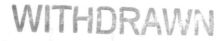

Also by Dr. Janet Starr Hull

*Sweet Poison: How the World's Most Popular Artificial Sweetener
    Is Killing Us – My Story*
10 Steps To Detoxification
Dr. Richardson's Alternative Cancer Diet

Visit Dr. Hull's website and sign up for her free health newsletter:

http://www.janethull.com

Also visit Dr. Hull's Splenda websites for updates, safe-sugar-free
recipes and more.

http://www.splendaexposed.com
http://www.issplendasafe.com

Splenda®
Is It Safe Or Not?

by
Janet Starr Hull, PhD, CN

with
Lynn Townsend Dealey

The Pickle Press
Dallas, Texas

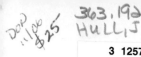
Copyright © 2004 by Janet Starr Hull, Ph.D., CN

Dr. Janet Starr Hull
P.O. Box 971
McKinney, TX 75070-0971

ISBN: 0-9771843-0-7

Hull, Janet Starr
        Splenda: Is It Safe or Not?

Jacket Cover and Interior Graphics: Lynn Townsend Dealey
http://www.lynntownsenddealey.com

The Pickle Press
http://www.thepicklepress.com
Manufactured in the U.S.A.

DISCLAIMER

This book is based on my personal experiences and research, and reflects my perceptions of the past, present and future. All information presented in this book is the result of my personal research and collaboration with professional, academic, and government colleagues, internationally. The personalities, events, actions, and conversations portrayed within the book have been reconstructed from my memory, various legal records, letters, personal papers, and press accounts. Some names and events have been altered to protect the privacy of individuals. Events involving the characters happened as described; only minor details have been altered.

This book is for educational purposes only and not intended to be considered legal, medical, or any other professional service. The information provided is not a replacement for professional advice or care. If you require nutritional, medical, or other expert services, please seek appropriate professional care. The author, contributors, publisher and their employees are not liable or held accountable for any damages arising from or in association with the application of any information contained in this book.

TABLE OF CONTENTS

Appendices

AUTHOR'S NOTE

The question I hear most often these days: "Is Splenda better than aspartame and NutraSweet?" The answer: "Yes, but - _no_."

I hate to be the bad guy and throw a wet blanket over Splenda as I did with aspartame, historically found in NutraSweet/Equal®, but sucralose may have harmful effects, too. I am one of many concerned. Even though sucralose doesn't appear as damaging as aspartame and the potential side effects are initially less obvious, there is evidence that the chlorine can accumulate in the body and create negative health effects. I do not recommend using Splenda, or any diet sweetener, especially for those who are pregnant, for children under eighteen years of age, for the elderly, for those with bladder or kidney problems, for those trying to get pregnant, and particularly for men with infertility issues.

The dangers of aspartame are now widely known, but the risks of using Splenda are not as well documented. Primarily, the sucralose in Splenda does not penetrate the blood brain barrier as aspartame does, hence entering the brain and creating neurotoxic havoc at the brain center. But sucralose can adversely affect the body in several ways because it IS a chemical substance and not natural sugar.

It is important to educate yourself on the facts about Splenda, NutraSweet/Equal, and all sugar substitutes available on today's sugar-free market. In order to make a decision whether to use chemical sweeteners or not, you must have all the data, both good and bad. But it is hard for the general public to find. I have spent over fifteen years working with victims of aspartame because the truth and information about the dangers of aspartame and Equal has been quietly steered away from public access since the early 1970s.

It appears the same patterns with aspartame (NutraSweet/Equal) are repeating with sucralose (Splenda). Their corporate claims of product safety and research results are almost identical to those used by The NutraSweet Company. As you read the pages of this book, note the comparisons between the products, the corporations, and the marketing strategies. Maybe consumers can prevent possible damage to their health from sucralose sooner than they did with aspartame, which has affected the health and lives of millions of innocent people since it was introduced into the public food supply over twenty years ago.

I am aware of the fact that many Americans are weight conscious, Type I or II diabetic, and concerned with hyperactivity and depression. Artificial chemical sugar-substitutes have become a part of our modern world, and there is little hope they will "go away." With that reality in mind, I offer these thoughts:

1. Consumers need to know everything possible about chemical food additives in order to make an educated decision whether to use chemical sugar substitutes or not.
2. Chemical sweeteners may be at the root of many unexplained disease symptoms.
3. YOU be the judge whether to give these chemicals to your children or to use them during pregnancy.
4. Carefully consider whether using chemical food additives is wise if you are suffering from a present chronic disease.

According to researchers, there is no clear-cut evidence that sugar substitutes are even useful in weight reduction. On the contrary, there is evidence that these substances may stimulate appetite. Aspartame has been on the market for over two decades, and we are now facing an international obesity epidemic among over 60 percent of both adults and children.

I have included research reports that demonstrate sucralose in Splenda has <u>not been proven</u> safe for long-term use. (Remember, many pharmaceuticals approved as "safe," have been taken off the market today.)

The research reports cite recurring laboratory results of infertility and gastrointestinal problems as a result of using sucralose. Aspartame research revealed lesions (holes) in the brains of laboratory rats, dead fetuses, cancer, and lower IQs. Didn't hear much about that, did you? Independent research results can be successfully played down and forgotten over time. I hope the facts provided within this book will stand strong and that people will remember that sucralose, as well as aspartame, has not been truly proven safe for the public food supply. At least you, the consumer, deserve to be informed about the "other side" of this safety issue so you can make up your own mind whether to use sucralose or not.

Wishing you all the best in good health, and may this book enlighten your nutritional education with new information concerning the artificial sweeteners flooding the modern marketplace.

To Your Health,

Janet Hull

CHAPTER 1

Splenda: Is It Safe Or Not?

Before you tear open that little yellow packet of sweetener and stir it into your coffee, please read this chapter, even if that's all you read.

Do you want to:

1. Avoid certain diseases and maintain health and vitality well into your later years?
2. Save your children from a slow poisoning from hidden toxins in their food?
3. Discover scientific data about overlooked poisons in your everyday life?
4. Avoid those vague health symptoms of illness that puzzle your doctor?
5. Be informed with inside information that mainstream media won't tell you?
6. Have control over your health through knowledge?
7. Desire to enjoy your grandchildren (and great-grandchildren)?
8. Not allow advertisers to "teach" you what's good for you?

Interested? Then we need to talk about a *sweetener war* sweeping across America. Perhaps you can sip on that cup of coffee <u>black</u> until we straighten out the confusing selection of artificial sweeteners out there. This book is a tool to protect your health – and your children's health – from a hidden danger that marketing experts have packaged attractively and seductively. You'll be shocked at what the "quiet side" of scientific research reveals.

It's time to admit that there is no free ticket to eating all the sugar-free products you desire without paying the high price of harming your body in the long run. The "technology of foods" (artificial sweeteners and manmade foods) has gone too far, and will not secure eternal health, beauty, slimness, or youth. <u>Laboratory chemicals are not the answer.</u>

Within the chapters of this book, I show you the evidence strongly suggesting that these chemical sweeteners could be harmful to your health. I reveal the government documents confirming saccharin (the pink packet) has always been safe, and illustrate how research on the chemical sweeteners aspartame and sucralose has been selectively presented to reflect positive findings.

As an educated consumer, you have a <u>choice</u>. You can protect yourself from <u>avoidable</u> illnesses by simply being aware of the sweet deception surrounding you. This book will "wake you up" more than that mug of java you're holding. But don't despair – there are plenty of <u>safe</u> alternatives to keep life "sweet."

The Sweetener Wars

The past twenty years a war has been going on in your own backyard. It's an escalating sweetener war. A battle for your dollar to satisfy an ever demanding "sweet tooth." It started in the United States, but has spread worldwide. Thousands of people have been injured, and hundreds have probably lost their lives. It's a battle of health versus business success, and I have uncovered the documents to show it.

Medical doctors, holistic doctors, nutritionists, journalists, researchers, and professors – many people have fought for the truth about the dangers of artificial sweeteners. In this unseen battle, these men and women you do not know have been fighting to protect you and your children from injury and possible death. With more new chemical sweeteners on the market today, the battle is far from being won.

After twenty years of NutraSweet/Equal® (aspartame) dominating the sweetener market, people are realizing for themselves that aspartame really is a foul food chemical, tragically harmful to their health. But the corporations deny there is a connection between aspartame and epidemic obesity, mental disturbances, addictions, and disease. They have left the proof to the consumer, who is now *getting the picture,* but at great personal cost. And the corporations work against the thousands of claims of bodily harm and death connected to artificial sweeteners.

Now, people may think Johnson & Johnson's Splenda, made from sucralose, has "come to the rescue" as the newest chemical sugar replacement "made from real sugar." People don't want to hear that it may be just as dangerous as aspartame, and this "white knight" of sweeteners is no improvement. I have listed documents that put the safety of this sweetener into question.

New chemical sweeteners (like Splenda) and the sweetener blends (aspartame, sucralose and acesulfame K blended together in one product) may be causing users to show signs of weight gain, disruption of sleep patterns, sexual dysfunction, increases in cancer, MS, Lupus, diabetes, and a list of epidemic degenerative diseases. The corporations continue to stand tough in their denial of any connection to chemical sweetener additives.

> **Never Enough: Artificial Sweeteners Create An Artificial Need**
> People forget that originally, sweetness was actually a by-product of food: nature's way to encourage living creatures to consume nutritious foods. Forced sweetness, revved-up sweetness, and artificial sweetness - all altered foods - are a trap that addict people to sweeter tastes.

Artificial sweeteners are marketed as having "more sweetness with no penalty of weight gain." People with eating disorders, children who are first learning about healthy food habits, diabetics and those with degenerative illnesses are being seduced by advertising campaigns touting that these chemicals are not only safe, but beneficial to human health. "And the added plethora of laboratory chemicals are entirely unnecessary to put in the public food supply," says Kelly Goyen, CEO of Empirical Labs.

"We've done a great job of redefining sweetness, and it's great to see it pay off," says Anne Rewey, Splenda marketing director for Ft. Washington, Pennsylvania-based McNeil. "We're committed to the leadership position in this market."

According to the Conference of the American College of Physicians *"we are talking about a plague of neurological diseases caused by these deadly poisons." (aspartame, sucralose, acesulfame-K)*

What Are Artificial Sweeteners and Why Are They Harmful?

Artificial sweeteners are a mix of unnatural chemicals combined in a laboratory that the body can't process. Basically, these chemicals either accumulate in your vital organs (*causing severe damage later*), pollute your bloodstream (*causing severe damage later*), or form the basis for eventual mutations of your cells (*causing severe damage later*).

Nature Versus Manmade: The Key To "Safe" Food
In a nutshell, whatever nature creates for food is usually safe for your body: whatever man creates for food (in the laboratory) may not be accepted by your body and can result in illness. Our bodies are like machines (only natural) that operate today just as they did thousands of years ago. They don't "understand" manmade chemicals and cannot fully process them. Forcing "foreign" materials into your body is like pouring shampoo into your car's gas tank: it wasn't meant to process it, so the engine stalls and stops working. As in a car, the chemical by-products pollute the system.

Which Artificial Sweeteners To Avoid?

- Sucralose (Splenda)
- Aspartame (NutraSweet/Equal®)
- Acesulfame-K (Sunett®)
- Neotame®
- Alitame®
- Cyclamate

Clever Advertising: What Was "Harmful" Yesterday Can Be "Hidden" Today!

Diet RC® cola was the first U.S. product with sucralose introduced in May 1998 with the tagline "No Aspartame" on the can. Nowadays, the tagline has been dropped and is no longer on the can because sucralose is now found blended with aspartame in numerous products such as The Coca-Cola Company's new C2 Coke®.

Is Saccharin Still Safe?

Saccharin, in my opinion, remains the safest of all the artificial sweeteners despite the misleading report twenty years ago that saccharin causes cancer. Its simplicity may be the key to its ability to be used by the body as a sugar substitute. Saccharin is not a "chemically combined" sweetener like the other artificial sweeteners, and is the safest choice for diabetics.

If you get confused on which colored packet sweetener is what, remember this good rule-of-thumb: Color Matters!

- The yellow packet (Splenda) = *caution* like in a traffic light
- The blue packet (Equal) = makes you feel *blue*
- The pink packet (Sweet'N'Low® or generic saccharin*) = you're in the *pink*!

What Are Safe Natural Sweeteners?

1. Stevia*
2. Raw, unprocessed sugar (Sucanat®)
3. Brown Rice Syrup
4. Barley Malt
5. Date Sugar
6. Honey
7. Maple Syrup

8. Molasses
9. Sorghum

*Safe for diabetics. Stevia is similar to saccharin – use it sparingly or it is bitter – otherwise, it's *naturally* delicious and a much healthier choice!

Secondary Natural Sweetener Choices (Use With Discretion)

1. Fructose
2. Fruit Juice Concentrate
3. Juice Concentrate
4. Sugar alcohols (Polyols)
   - Isomalt
   - Lactitol
   - Malitol
   - Mannitol
   - Sorbitol
   - Xylitol
5. Turbinado® Sugar
6. Tagatose

What Exactly Is Splenda?

Splenda is the trade name for sucralose, a relatively new manmade, artificial sweetener. Johnson & Johnson bought the rights in 1998 to sell sucralose in the United States as Splenda. Its basic characteristics are:

- Its taste is nearly identical to sugar because it's made from sugar
- Its "trademark" inability to break down in processing or in storage

Why is Splenda potentially harmful?

It contains chlorine, which is a carcinogen. The Splenda marketers insist it is chemically "bound" so it cannot be "released" in the body during digestion. I question that, and wonder if this artificial chemical can safely pass through the human body. Wait until you read what chlorine can do to the body. You decide if you want to ingest this chemical.

Sucralose (Splenda) is a chlorocarbon - a chlorine-containing compound. The chlorocarbons have long been known for causing organ, genetic, and reproductive damage. It should be no surprise, then, that testing of sucralose revealed organ, genetic, and reproductive damage. Research on lab rats showed up to forty percent shrinkage of the thymus gland, a gland that is the very foundation of our immune system. The contamination of water supplies by chlorocarbons is a serious problem in most European countries today, making many people very ill. Due to the chlorine content in Splenda, sucralose can cause inflammation and swelling of the liver and kidneys, in addition to calcification of the kidney, as shown in animal studies. If you experience kidney pain, cramping, or an irritated bladder after using sucralose, stop using it immediately.

> Sucralose is patented as a manmade "chlorinated sucrose sweetener" and it is registered as "chlorinated sucrose." Chlorinated sucrose is not found anywhere in nature, like real sugar (sucrose) that is extracted from sugar cane and sugar beets. Chlorinated sucrose exists because of man.

Why is chlorine harmful? Doesn't it kill germs in my tap water?

Let's digress for a moment: Manmade chlorine (found in Splenda) is essentially bleach. There is natural chlorine found

<u>in nature, but it is totally different from Splenda's laboratory invention.</u>

First, let's see what OSHA (the Federal Occupational Safety and Hazard Association) says in its regulations for manmade chlorine, the chemical used in Splenda.

OSHA States: Any animal that eats or drinks chlorine (especially on a regular basis) is at risk of cancer. *The Merck Manuel and OSHA 40 SARA 120 Hazardous Waste Handbook* states that chlorine is a carcinogen and emergency procedures should be taken when exposed by swallowing, inhaling, or contact through the skin. Currently, the safety of chlorine added to our public water supply is being questioned as a cause of cancer. (More on chlorine in the public water supply in Chapter Two.)

Whenever I think about chlorine, I remember a sobering experience I had in 1987 with chlorine when I was a Hazardous Waste and Emergency Response engineer:

Mr. Jones, a Texas rancher west of Dallas, called the office in a panic. He'd bought an additional 2,000 acres adjacent to his ranch and discovered an old building on the property. "It has five huge ole' unmarked drums full of some sort of liquid," he said. "They don't smell right; smells like chlorine to me. I have cattle and I know that stuff can kill 'em."

I was part of the Emergency Hazardous Waste Response Team at Environmental Engineering and Geotechnics (EE&G) at the time, and we were called out to investigate. Whenever unmarked storage drums are discovered, an OSHA certified emergency response team (HAZWOPER team) is called on the scene to safely remove and dispose of the unidentified material.

As usual, it was a hot Texas summer day, but it felt even hotter when I was sealed tightly in my biohazard suit and oxygen tank. It was as if I were in a zip-lock baggie - not one centimeter of flesh can be exposed - my eyes, nose and lungs were fully protected from vapors, and I whispered a quick prayer before I entered the area, hoping nothing blew up in my face.

Step by step, our three-man team slowly inched toward the drums. We each carried long white sticks to carefully probe each drum at first contact. If they were going to explode, it would be at the first tap. We carried no beepers, no cell phones, no walkie-talkies, watches or any devices that could trigger a spark.

When we cautiously pried the lid off the first drum, it hissed and we instinctively shut our eyes and pursed our lips. No explosion.

Removing tiny glass vials from our supply kit, we dipped the sample containers into the green liquid inside each drum and walked them over to the chemist waiting outside the quarantine area. His "field chemistry" performed on the samples confirmed the drums were filled with chorine. If we had not been protected with airtight suits, our lungs could have been scarred and our systems poisoned from the vapors, because manufactured chlorine is a dangerous poison.

We called the proper authorities, filled out our government paperwork, and high-tailed it out of there, leaving the chlorine disposal to the next trained team.

If those drums had spilled, we would have evacuated within a five-mile radius, tested the surrounding soil and downstream groundwater for chlorine periodically over the next eighteen months, and notified all the neighbors within a ten-mile radius of possible carcinogenic exposure to livestock, animals, and humans.

Manufactured chlorine is an extremely toxic biohazard, and I was shocked when I first learned chlorine is in Splenda.

So, feel like munching on a few sugar-free cookies made with sucralose about now? What are the guarantees that this poisonous chlorine chemical <u>won't</u> break down in your extremely efficient digestive system – a complex machine with seven organs all valiantly trying to break it down for absorption? After all, your body thinks that's why you ate it, right? So chances are, it can be digested and assimilated into your body to some degree. As with aspartame, after people get ill, will we hear another resounding "oops!" from the industry and "I told you so" from independent scientists? Why take the chance?

<u>What about table salt (sodium chloride)? Isn't that a "good" chlorine?</u>

Again, this is manmade chlorine, not nature's chlorine. Natural chlorine occurs in the soil, spring water, and in foods, and it is relatively harmless. As usual, any created laboratory chemical is questionable for human consumption. Read on!

A study by Dr. Niels Skakkebaek of the University of Copenhagen demonstrated that the average human sperm counts have dropped in Denmark by almost fifty percent due to the presence of manmade chlorine found within human tissues and breast milk.

"People consume chlorine every day in foods like melon, tomatoes, lettuce, and mushrooms as well as prepared products such as peanut butter," says Dr. Leslie Goldsmith, Vice President, Safety and Science Affairs, McNeil Nutritionals, in a letter she sent to me.

It seems that when people refer to chlorine, even Dr. Goldsmith, they don't realize the difference between nature's version of chlorine and man's. Those vegetables contain natural chlorine – not manmade chlorine. All chlorine is not the same. It's really that simple. (NutraSweet representatives also stated the exact same thing about the manmade methanol in aspartame - that it's in our food, anyway.)

<u>So, is table salt (sodium chloride) a natural form of chlorine?</u>

No. You don't need **salt** in your diet at all. You need **sodium** – the element found in nature. Man created the "sodium chloride" concept.

<u>You can eat all the table salt you want and your cells can still be sodium deficient.</u> Getting your sodium from plants rather than from table salt is the better choice to make. It has been proven that sodium from plants will not cause high blood pressure. Not only does table salt contribute to high blood pressure and hardening of the arteries, but it also stimulates unnecessary swelling in the cells of the body and overworks the heart. When your doctor warns you to "watch your salt," that means to stop using sodium chloride, but your body still needs *sodium*. So, eat your kale and spinach and dark greens. It will keep your arteries young and elastic, help your blood flow more efficiently to rejuvenate your organs, and even your sense of smell will improve significantly.

Weird Science: How Splenda Was Discovered

It seems that most of the artificial sweeteners have been discovered by accident, and sucralose is no exception. This is *yet another* strange "fortuitous discovery" of *yet another* chemical sweetener.

In 1976, Tate & Lyle, a British sugar company, was searching for ways to blend sucrose (sugar) with laboratory chemicals. In collaboration with Professor Leslie Hough's laboratory at Queen's College in London, halogenated sugars were currently being tested. Responding to a request for "testers" for these experimental chlorinated sugars, foreign graduate student Shashikant Phadnis signed up for "taste tests." His participation in the research project led to the discovery that chlorinated sugars are sweet and have potencies hundreds to thousands of times greater than sugar.

Excited about their new discovery, the manufacturers of Splenda have been spreading the word about their new sweetener, but they do admit real sugar (unprocessed sucrose) is better for the body than sweeteners from the laboratory:

"Sucralose is made from sugar, but is derived from sucrose (sugar) through a process that selectively substitutes three atoms of chlorine for three hydrogen-oxygen groups on the sucrose molecule. No artificial sweetener made in the laboratory is going to be neither natural to the body nor safer than unprocessed sugar," they state.

The Tate & Lyle study was originally investigating the sweetness of sugar spin-offs, specifically those substituted with halogens. Halogens are powerful elements that help dissolve one substance into another. The researchers at Queen's College determined that five closely related halogens - fluorine, chlorine, bromine, iodine, and astatine (see below) - change the sweetness of the sugar molecule, with chlorine and bromine being the most effective.

The Halogens:

1. Fluorine - poisonous pale yellow gas

2. Chlorine - poisonous pale green gas
3. Bromine - toxic and caustic brown volatile liquid
4. Iodine - shiny black solid which forms an inspiringly beautiful violet vapor when heated
5. Astatine – (means unstable) a manmade radioactive chemical that does not occur in nature

Chlorine was chosen because as a lighter halogen, it more easily dissolves in other substances, and combines readily with the sucrose for sugar substitution. The chlorine has to be chemically altered, though, to be very tightly bound so that it doesn't break down inside the human body.

Food For Thought:
If the chorine in sucralose breaks free before it is completely excreted from your body, doesn't it make the contents of sucralose a carcinogen because chlorine causes cancer in humans and animals?

Canada became the first country to approve the use of Splenda in 1991, and the US Food and Drug Administration (FDA) granted American marketing approval in 1998. Johnson & Johnson purchased the rights to develop sucralose in the United States as a commercially available product. They created an individual company, McNeil Specialty Products (renamed McNeil Nutritionals), as a part of the Johnson & Johnson corporate umbrella for the exclusive purpose of marketing the new sucralose product "Splenda" in 2000.

How Do They Make Splenda?

Splenda (sucralose) is created in the lab, using a complex process involving dozens of chemicals you and I can barely pronounce - let alone consume. Basically, the chemists force chlorine into an unnatural chemical bond with a sugar molecule, resulting in a sweeter product, but at a price: a huge amount of artificial chemicals must be added to keep sucralose from digesting in our bodies. These toxic substances also prevent (hopefully) the dangerous chlorine molecules from detaching from the sugar molecule inside the digestive system, which would be a carcinogenic hazard.

To illustrate the alarming "chemical soup" required to create sucralose, I have listed here the actual process for producing this sweetener. I highlighted the chemicals in bold type for emphasis. According to the Splenda International Patent A23L001-236 and PEP Review #90-1-4 (July 1991), sucralose is synthesized by this five-step process:

1. Sucrose is tritylated with **trityl chloride** in the presence of **dimethylformamide** and **4-methylmorpholine** and the tritylated sucrose is then acetylated with **acetic anhydride**,
2. The resulting TRISPA (6,1',6'-tri-O-trityl-penta-O-acetylsucrose) is chlorinated with **hydrogen chloride** in the presence of **toluene**,
3. The resulting 4-PAS (sucrose 2,3,4,3',4'-pentaacetate) is heated in the presence of **methyl isobutyl ketone** and **acetic acid**,
4. The resulting 6-PAS (sucrose 2,3,6,3',4'-pentaacetate) is chlorinated with **thionyl chloride** in the presence of **toluene** and **benzyltriethylammonium chloride**, and
5. The resulting TOSPA (sucralose pentaacetate) is treated with **methanol** (wood alcohol, a poison) in the presence of **sodium methoxide** to produce sucralose.

The Splenda marketers stress that sucralose is *"made from sugar but is derived from this sugar through a process that selectively substitutes three atoms of chlorine for three hydrogen-oxygen groups on the sucrose molecule."* While this is true, it is a deceptively simple description, implying that sucralose is just a <u>benign sugar with a touch of chlorine</u>, and thereby, safe for consumption. According to research on the hydrolysis of sugars, just the process of inserting chlorine into the sugar molecule (hydrolysis means breaking it into smaller molecules) ultimately allows these chemicals to penetrate the intestinal wall.

So sucralose becomes a "low-calorie" sugar with a complicated process that results in Splenda's chemical formal: 1,6-dichloro-1, 6-dideoxy-BETA-D-fructofuranosyl-4-chloro-4-deoxy-alpha-D-galactopyranoside. (See Appendix I.)

<u>*This is Splenda.*</u> They say it is a perfectly safe sugar molecule.

More Hidden Chemicals In Splenda

Did you know if a product includes an ingredient that is a proven carcinogen but is less than two percent of its total chemical make-up, it does not have to be listed as an ingredient, nor does it have to be tested for product safety or **labeled as a carcinogen**? Just as an example, a food product could have 2.5 percent rat poison as a minor ingredient, but does not have to name the rat poison on the ingredient list. With the number of chemicals used in manufacturing food products today, the ingredient lists would probably be too long to fit on any of the labels, needless to say.

The FDA states in their Final Report on Splenda that sucralose is "produced at an approximate purity of ninety-eight percent." (See Appendices II and III for the full FDA Final Reports on Splenda and acesulfame-K.) The other two percent does not have to be reported to the FDA, nor listed as added ingredients. *So what's in the other two percent?*

1. Acetone
2. Acetic acid

3. Acetyl alcohol
4. Acetic anhydride
5. Ammonium chloride
6. Benzene
7. Chlorinated sulfates
8. Ethyl alcohol
9. Isobutyl ketones
10. Formaldehyde
11. Hydrogen chloride
12. Lithium chloride
13. Methanol
14. Sodium methoxide
15. Sulfuryl chloride
16. Trityl chloride
17. Toluene
18. Thionyl chloride

Although manufacturing guidelines specify limits on these hidden substances, there are no assurances these limits have been met since they do not have to be reported. In addition, the FDA does not presently require an Environmental Impact Statement for sucralose, so it's open season for the rules, at present.

Now you can see why I do not recommend sucralose for pregnancy or for children, especially after reading this list.

Is Splenda Digested Or Not?

Because of their patented multi-step process, corporate marketers insist the body doesn't recognize Splenda as a sugar, a carbohydrate, or "anything," so it doesn't metabolize it AT ALL. I disagree.

The only way sucralose can be prevented from breaking down and passing through the intestinal wall is to be altered into a substance the body doesn't recognize, and that requires using the myriad of chemicals listed previously.

Ingesting these grossly-mutated molecules can create tremendous stress in the body. Many people complain of stomach cramping, bloating or diarrhea from using sucralose. More bladder infections, blood in the urine, kidney problems, and accompanying lower backache have appeared since both aspartame and sucralose came onto the market. The number of pharmaceutical sales for bladder control, recurring bladder infections, and kidney disease support this connection, as do the hundreds of case histories I receive daily from people whose symptoms vanish when they stop using sucralose, aspartame, and blends of chemical sweeteners.

> NOTE: An individual's reaction to sucralose and other artificial sweeteners depends upon how much is used and how often, past and current health status, and the degree of other toxins present inside the body.

Yet, Splenda representatives are aggressively pushing sucralose into the international market and defending its safety as completely risk-free to human health.

"Sucralose is harmless, poorly absorbed, and does not accumulate in the body. There is absolutely no need for concern about the safety of sucralose due to the chlorine molecules used in its manufacture," states Dr. Leslie Goldsmith of McNeil Nutritionals.

Again, I disagree. Laboratory chlorine is laboratory chlorine. Replacing natural sugar with chlorine can be harmful.

If You Have A Healthy Digestive System, You Just Might Digest Splenda

How do you know that you would or wouldn't digest the chlorine in Splenda? How does McNeil know? Every human being is unique.

We forget the whole purpose of eating: human beings require food to grow, reproduce, and maintain good health. Foods are *supposed* to digest to provide fuel for survival. The human digestive system is amazing, and it will do anything to assimilate what you give it to support life. And you're trying to fool it when you feed it fake foods.

The breakdown of a diet cola is achieved through a combination of mechanical and enzymatic processes. To accomplish this breakdown, the digestive tract uses a team effort, requiring considerable assistance from the digestive organs such as the salivary glands, the liver, and pancreas, which dump their secretions into the digestive tract system. Without the pancreatic enzymes, you would starve from lack of nutrients and become malnourished.

In many ways, the digestive system is like a well-run engine where a large number of complex tasks take place. Look how many major organs are dedicated to digestion alone:

1. Mouth
2. Esophagus
3. Stomach
4. Liver
5. Pancreas
6. Small Intestine
7. Large Intestine

It is unlikely sucralose can escape this arduous journey through your body without breaking down in some way. If your body is digesting properly, *resistance is futile.*

In fact, research shows that artificial sweeteners can create a fatty liver. The liver enzymes are elevated because the body is working so hard to digest something it doesn't understand.

Conflicting Reports About Splenda's Absorption In The Body

With all this information on the dangers of aspartame - and now sucralose - who do we believe – the corporations, the government, researchers, or consumers? According to the FDA's "Final Rule" report, eleven to twenty-seven percent of sucralose is absorbed in the human body, and the remainder is excreted unchanged in the fecal waste. According to the Japanese Food Sanitation Council, as much as forty percent of ingested sucralose is absorbed. According to the creators of sucralose, Tate & Lyle, fifteen percent is absorbed. According to McNeil Nutritionals, marketers of Splenda, zero percent is absorbed. Who do we believe?

The FDA also states in their final report, "Because sucralose may hydrolyze in some food products...the resulting hydrolysis products may also be ingested by the consumer." They also report that there is some concern about tumor growth in certain studies with mice, and many of the other tests submitted have "inconclusive" results. (See Appendix II FDA Final Rule Report – Sucralose.)

Toxicologist Judith Bellin reviewed studies on rats starved under experimental conditions, and concluded that their growth rate was reduced by as much as a third without the thymus losing a significant amount of weight (less than seven percent). The changes were much more obvious in rats fed sucralose. While the animals' growth rate was reduced by between seven and twenty percent, their thymus glands shrank by as much as forty percent.

The absorbed levels of sucralose were found in laboratory studies to concentrate in the liver, kidney, and gastrointestinal tract of laboratory animals. Understanding how digestion works, now we know why.

Research animals fed sucralose exhibited the following symptoms:

1. Unexplained death
2. Shrunken thymus glands (up to forty percent shrinkage)
3. Enlarged liver and kidneys
4. Atrophy of lymph follicles in the spleen and thymus
5. Reduced growth rate
6. Decreased white blood cell count
7. Hyperplasia of the pelvis
8. Extension of the pregnancy period
9. Aborted pregnancy
10. Decreased fetal body weight and placental weights
11. Chronic diarrhea
12. Maternal gastrointestinal disturbances

> **What's Good For the Rat Is Good For the Human**
> McNeil representatives state negative animal study results
> do not apply to human sucralose consumption, as decreased
> interest in the artificial sweetness throughout several studies
> was found to only occur in the rat studies. (The rats stopped
> eating.) The decreased taste pleasure led to decreased thymus
> weight "only in the rats."
>
> So why do they do studies on rats, then? Are they saying that
> only positive lab results apply to human product safety, and
> negative results don't count? If all the studies on rats attempt
> to prove safety for humans, aren't the studies proving
> significant danger as well?

Totally And Completely Harmless?

McNeil Nutritionals markets sucralose as flawlessly safe for
everyone. They claim it has been repeatedly tested so they can
prove it is completely harmless. Nothing is totally and completely
harmless. They also claim that sucralose is the most tested food
additive in history. I quote, "...more than one-hundred studies
on the safety of sucralose designed to meet the highest scientific
standards have been conducted and evaluated over the course of
twenty years." Having worked with the aspartame issue over the
past thirteen years, I know this statement is debatable.

McNeil representatives state: "Millions of people have safely
enjoyed Splenda and products made with sucralose since its
introduction more than ten years ago. It is one of the most
tested food ingredients ever introduced and its safety has
been confirmed by regulatory authorities in more than sixty
countries."

They also said the same thing about aspartame, which had

over <u>200</u>-documented research studies performed by both corporations and independent researchers. Don't be fooled by the numbers. In my opinion, a large number of studies usually implies negative results that require more scrutiny. I am suspicious of a product that claims to be safe if an inordinate number of tests are run. To me, this implies negative results that must be retested.

Consumers are witnessing the same pattern with sucralose as with aspartame in so many ways. There are comparisons between sucralose and aspartame research and marketing throughout this book. I'm noticing that Splenda's developmental strategy is similar to aspartame's, which I discussed in my first book, <u>Sweet Poison</u>: no long-term studies by the manufacturers have been done on humans; researchers employed by these companies were responsible for the results submitted to the FDA, to the media, and to scientific journals; only selective results were reported (out of the *hundreds* of experiments performed); and "government/ corporate involvement" is clearly documented.

Safe And Natural

The corporations maintain sucralose is safe and natural. We must remember that independent research results are just as valid as those funded by the corporations who make the product in question.

"While there are a lot of industry-sponsored safety studies on these substances, I don't believe there is enough independent research to tell us whether we should be using them in moderation or at all," said Dr. Jeanette Newton Keith, a gastroenterologist and an assistant professor of medicine at The University of Chicago's Pritzker School of Medicine.

In the absence of independent data, she advises patients to avoid the non-nutritive sweeteners entirely. She accredits anecdotal reports linking aspartame (Equal®) to memory loss, seizures, chronic headaches and neurological disorders. After years of personally working with hundreds of patients suffering from aspartame poisoning, I agree with Dr. Keith and encourage all practitioners to consider artificial sweeteners as a contributing cause of illness, especially when their doctor cannot offer any known cause for observable health symptoms.

Baking With Splenda

"Baking studies have shown that Splenda is exceptionally heat-stable," state McNeil representatives. "No measurable breakdown of Splenda occurred in any of the baked goods tested. One hundred percent of sucralose was recovered from cakes, biscuits, and crackers after baking at typical temperatures of 350°F, 410°F, and 450°F, respectively." Splenda studies prove that Splenda maintains its sweetness during cooking and in storage for long periods of time.

Barndt and Jackson, a research team, performed one such study in 1990. The purpose of the "sucralose processing study" was to demonstrate sucralose stability in a variety of common baked goods. Yellow cake, cookies, and graham crackers were selected because they represent a common cross-section of common ingredients and typical process conditions used in the baking industry. For each baked product, no peaks other than sucralose could be detected. Using aqueous/methanolic (methanol) extracts of the baked products, a one-hundred percent sucralose recovery was found, which proved sucralose did not interact with any other ingredients during baking, and that the compound remained stable under baking conditions. Its inability to break down when heated also proves it maintains extremely unnatural physical properties both in baked food products and in the human body.

Kim Clay, director of communications for Merisant Corp., the current Chicago-based manufacturer of NutraSweet/Equal®, was quoted as admitting that Equal not used well in baking, "There are special recipes that the Equal test kitchen has developed, so Equal can be used in baking," Clay explained. "You just have to do it a certain way, at the end of the baking cycle."

> So, Equal doesn't bake safely and Splenda doesn't "bake" at all - what is this doing to the health of a five year old?

Splenda is marketed as being 600 times sweeter than sugar, but its sweetness can vary up to 4,000 times sweeter according to the patent information, and depending on the food application it is found in and what other artificial sweeteners it is blended with. And the "bigger the number" doesn't mean it's necessarily better. The more inflated a chemical sweetener is (such as 600 times or 4,000 times sweeter than real sugar), the farther from natural it is, the more chemicals are required to prevent it from "digesting" which makes it harmful to the body, and the harder it is to cook with.

"What most people don't know," comments Kelly Goyen, CEO of Empirical Labs, "is sweeteners merely fifty to one hundred times sweeter than sugar bake better and retain more of the texture of real food. And to enhance sucralose's sweeter taste, it is bulked-up with maltodextrin, a starchy powder, so it can measure more like sugar."

> A basic law of physics: when any matter is heated, it breaks down. Then, how unnatural is a substance that doesn't break down when heated? I wouldn't want that in my cocoa!

Splenda's Shelf-Life

Results of a 1999 McNeil study of carbonated cola at pH 3.1 (very acidic) sweetened with either Splenda or aspartame, showed that after one year of storage at seventy-three degrees Fahrenheit, ninety-nine percent of the Splenda remained unchanged compared to twenty-nine percent of the aspartame. The effect of storage on the flavor of cola drinks sweetened with sugar (control group), sucralose, aspartame, and an aspartame/acesulfame K blend was studied over a period of six months in storage at twenty degrees Centigrade at pH 3.0.

Sucralose stability and flavor retention were of particular interest. An "expert sensory panel" confirmed each sweetener system to be of equal sweetness and comparable in flavor:

- The sucralose cola retained an initial flavor, except for a slight increase in metallic flavor, and maintained its approximate sweetness intensity over the duration of six months.
- In comparison, both other experimental sweeteners decreased in sweetness intensity and increased in bitterness.
- The sucralose cola retained its cola flavor over six months.
- Aspartame and aspartame/acesulfame-K blend colas decreased in cola flavor.
- The control sugar cola retained its initial flavor and sweetness.

So if sucralose is "indigestible" due to its laboratory compounding as the manufacturer claims, and corporate studies show it remains inert and almost completely unaltered after sitting in a can for six months, then we have yet another serious health problem to consider – the body by nature will work even more diligently to digest the chemicals, elevating liver enzymes, stomach enzymes, and intestinal bacteria – all placing stress and trauma on the body, and depleting its nutrients.

Are Artificial Sweeteners Safe For Children?

Have your kids been out of sorts lately? Do they complain of more frequent tummy aches, malaise, mood swings or aggression? Have you read the labels on what they are eating at home, at school, and away from the house?

"Consumption of even moderate amounts of aspartame during pregnancy may produce a dramatic increase in the number of children born with diminished brain function," warned Diana Dow-Edwards, PhD research scientist, SUNY Health Science Center, Brooklyn, NY. Dow-Edward's research began in the mid-1980s, but her early warnings of aspartame's harmful effects on fetuses during pregnancy have fallen upon deaf ears. With the rapid rise in mental illness amongst children, AD/HD and hyperactivity, depression, and lower IQs, why hasn't research such as Dow-Edward's been considered as a probable cause for rising mental disease among modern children? Why haven't mothers been warned that artificial sweeteners can cause birth defects and mental retardation if taken at the time of conception and early pregnancy?

> WARNING: Children are especially at risk for neurological disorders and should NOT be given aspartame and its blend with sucralose or acesulfame K.

I can relate many case histories of children having seizures and other mental disturbances while using NutraSweet®. Unfortunately, it is not always easy to convince a mother that aspartame is to blame for her child's illnesses. Only by trial and success will she be able to warn other mothers to take their children's health into their own hands.

Splenda manufacturers even admit: "One should note, however, that foods made with low-calorie sweeteners are not normally a recommended part of a child's diet, since calories are important to a growing child's body."

Pay attention to this statement.... *Children should not be encouraged to grow up on fake foods.* But just like cigarettes and alcohol: "do what I say and not what I do." And we wonder why the younger generation is angry, ill, and ridden with AD/HD, depression, hypoglycemia, and diabetes. How many kids do you see taking a sip of mom's diet cola or chewing a stick of sugar-free gum?

Children raised on chemical diets are more likely to develop physical and mental disorders, and as Dow-Edwards predicted, the evidence is surfacing at epidemic levels in America and other developed countries.

Chemical Toxicity: The Mounting Debt Our Bodies Will Pay

The modern day sweetener debate is part of an alarming trend worldwide – the subtle introduction of more and more chemical toxins into our food supply. From pesticides to hormones to steroids, antibiotics, preservatives, dyes, and now fake sugars – the list goes on and on.

During a 1990 conference in Brussels, the vice chair of the International Sweeteners Association (ISA) Public Relation's Committee Lesley Yeoman (of Tate & Lyle, creators of sucralose) stated, "Industry itself would like to see fewer regulations. We can't avoid the fact that sweeteners are classed as additives and regulated heavily. But the ISA's position is that this is unnecessary."

Richard Wurtman, MD, Director and neuroscientist at Massachusetts Institute of Technology (MIT), stated as early as 1987, " Aspartame is a synthetic compound. We should not try to imply that synthetic compounds have the same fate in the body as naturally occurring foods. The advertising is deceptive."

Interestingly in New Zealand in the summer of 2005, New Zealand Sugar lodged a complaint through the Advertising Standards Complaint Board against Splenda's marketers, Johnson & Johnson Pacific, for misleading advertising. The Panel ruled to uphold the complaint.

With the onslaught of illness and disease syndromes plaguing our modern world today, I'd say Wurtman has been proven correct over Yoeman.

The rapid increase of chemicals in our environment, food and medicine has greatly challenged the human body's ability to rid itself of toxins. Symptoms related to chemical toxicity vary from person to person as each person's body is individual, but one common symptom of toxicity is the breakdown of the human immune system. This response opens the gateway for various diseases in the body. Reactions to toxic chemicals found in artificial sweeteners can damage the nervous system, followed by anxiety, depression, increased nervousness, blood disorders, and hormone dysfunction.

Symptoms Of Chemical Toxicity:

A
Abnormal hardening of the bones
Accelerated aging
Aches and pains in bones and muscles (i.e. Fibromyalgia)
Allergies
Anemia
Angina

B
Birth defects
Behavioral changes
Blood problems
Blurred vision
Brain damage
Breathing problems

C
Cataracts
Colitis
Constipation
Cramping

D
Depression
Disorientation
Distractibility
Dizziness/vertigo
Dry skin and eyes

E
Eye damage

F
Fatigue/malaise
Fever/low-grade

H
Headaches/migraines
Hyperactivity/ADD-ADHD

I
Indigestion/acid reflux
Impulsiveness/OCD
Injury to cells
Insomnia
Irritability

L
Lack of concentration
Liver damage
Loss of appetite
Loss of hair
Loss of memory
Loss of libido
Lung damage

M
Metabolic problems
Mineral deficiencies

N
Nausea
Nerve disorders
Numbness
Neurological disorders

P
Protein/sugar in urine

S
Seizures
Sexual disorders
Skeletal malformation
Skin ailments/rashes

T
Tumors

V
Vitamin deficiencies

Patent Registration

When examining the patent information submitted for Splenda, some very interesting information surfaced that is not widely known. The information is technical, yet it is important to transcribe the data as it is written in the patent. (See Appendix III for the complete text.)

What do these reports reveal? In the Abstract for the International Patent, the company referred to Splenda as chlorinated sucrose, which we have already questioned as toxic. The corporation also lists toxic chemical compounds used in the chlorination of sucrose. When comparing the two CAS Registry Reports, not only do the additional chemicals used in formulating sucralose come to light, but there appear to be conflicts in the interpretation of data, as well.

One patent report records sucralose as being 600 times the sweetness of sugar, while a second patent report states sucralose as having the sweetening power four to 2000 times that of sugar. Mike R. Jenner, one of the inventors of sucralose, co-authored the report "History and Development of Sucralose" with Samuel V. Molinary. Molinary is the Research Director for PepsiCo and was the former Director of Scientific Affairs for GD Searle

Pharmaceuticals, owner of Monsanto Chemical Company and The NutraSweet Company. He is also Panel Co-Chairman of the International Life Sciences Institute (ILSI).

What Is The ILSI? As written on their website, ILSI, founded in 1978, "is a global network of scientists devoted to enhancing scientific basis for public *health decision-making.*" They work closely with the World Health Organization (WHO), and "receive the majority of their funding and financial support through government funding, corporations, and foundations throughout the world." Some of their members include:

- McNeil Nutritionals
- Tate & Lyle LTD
- The Coca-Cola Company
- Merisant Corporation
- Monsanto Chemical Company
- PepsiCo
- Abbot Laboratories
- Merck & Company
- Ajinomoto
- McDonalds
- The Kellogg Company
- Novartis
- The Kodak Company

(A complete list of members is included in Appendix IV.)

A detailed explanation of each of the chemicals involved in the processing of sucralose, along with the research supporting public health dangers are included in Chapter Eight, Research Studies.

Foreign Approval Of Splenda

The U.S. Food and Drug Administration, and the government food authority committees and the Health Ministries in Canada,

Mexico, Dominican Republic, Jamaica, Trinidad & Tobago, Argentina, and Brazil have confirmed the safety of sucralose. So have the countries of Colombia, Peru, Venezuela, Uruguay, Romania, Lebanon, Qatar, Bahrain, Pakistan, Tajikistan, China, South Africa, and Tanzania.

Re-read the list of these countries: Mexico, Jamaica, Tajikistan and Tanzania. These are the countries in which Splenda was first marketed, and the countries used as sites of approval.

These are wonderful countries with vivid cultures and interesting people, but these countries are not nations with the same lifestyle, technology, or mass marketing strategies compared to the United States'. These countries are more concerned with birth control, food staples, hostile take-over, and drought - not diet sweeteners, weight loss campaigns, and soft drink machines placed in every business and school. Let's compare apples to apples. Their bodies are not saturated with the same chemicals as high-tech, First World countries. Results will differ with lifestyle/chemical exposures.

FDA Approval

Dr. Adrian Gross was the FDA toxicologist who tried to stop NutraSweet's "second" approval attempt for aspartame. He told Congress that aspartame violated the Delaney Amendment that forbids putting anything in food that was suspect of causing cancer. He said that *beyond any shadow of a doubt, aspartame could cause brain tumors and brain cancer.* Because of this, he told Congress they shouldn't be able to set an allowable daily intake. His last words to Congress will always be remembered, " ... and if the FDA violates its own law, who is left to protect the public?"

As stated in the Delaney Clause [section 409(c)(3)(A) of the act], "...no food additive shall be deemed to be safe if it is found to induce cancer when ingested by man or animal." But a loophole exists.

As the FDA states in the Final Rule report for the artificial sweetener acesulfame K:

> "The Delaney clause applies to the additive itself and not to constituents used to process the additive. Thus, where an additive has not been shown to cause cancer, even though it contains a carcinogenic impurity, the additive is not subject to the legal effect of the Delaney Clause. Rather, the additive is properly evaluated under the general safety standard using risk assessment procedures to determine whether there is a reasonable certainty that no harm will result from the proposed use of the additive [Scott v. FDA, 728 F.2d 322 (6th Cir. 1984)]."

Therefore, even though the ingredients methanol and chlorine used to make aspartame and sucralose, respectively, are proven carcinogens, they are not considered as such according to the final product safety rulings for aspartame and sucralose.

Dr. Jacqueline Verett, a second FDA toxicologist, told Congress in 1981 that "all aspartame studies were built on a foundation of sand and should be thrown out." It's all a matter of public record.

Has the FDA repeated the aspartame approval process for sucralose, allowing a product with proven carcinogens to flood our food supply? Only time will tell, as it has with aspartame. Yet, at the cost of human health.

Knowledge is power. As an educated consumer, you have the awareness to choose what you and your family will ingest. Unnatural artificial sweeteners may affect your health. Why take the chance? With this book, you woke up and smelled the coffee just in time. Now you can drink it safely.

CHAPTER 2

Chlorine: In Your Swimming Pool And In Your Diet Cola

The inventors of Splenda admit around fifteen percent of sucralose is absorbed by the body, but they <u>cannot</u> guarantee you (out of this fifteen percent) what amount of chlorine stays in your body and what percent flushes out.

So, do you feel lucky today as you sprinkle that yellow packet of powder in your tea? You may be alarmed once you realize how chlorine (in that packet), this common chemical we've trusted as a "purifier," can actually affect our health in more ways than you know. Hopefully, this chapter will help you hesitate before you let your toddler take another sip of your diet cola.

Chlorine Is A Carcinogen And More

Manmade/manufactured chlorine is a known carcinogen and can be harmful to all living things. Zoologists, biologists and environmental engineers continually witness chlorine's devastating effects on plants and animals. The deformities in bird eggs and reptile eggs, mutations of frogs and lizards, infertility and birth defects, and even cancer in wild animals are well-documented effects on wildlife due to man's heavy use of chlorine.

But some corporations claim that the effects of chlorine on humans are different—that somehow we are exempt from harm. They maintain that chlorine, and the other toxic chemicals used in products such as Splenda, do not harm humans in any way. They market these toxic food chemicals as totally flawless and one-hundred percent safe for human health.

Contrary to what marketers may say, human beings are not "exempt" from these harmful effects of chlorine. Chlorine does bioaccumulate*, and most animals are showing signs of physical harm because of it. We have yet to know what the long-term effects of chlorine in our foods will be on humans.

*Note: Bioaccumulation refers to the accumulation of a substance in a living organism as a result of its intake both in the food and from the environment. Determination of the B-factor (Bioaccumulation Factor) is extremely important in the risk analysis of any compound.

Why Is Chlorine So "Bad" All Of A Sudden?

It's simple: Because of the overuse of chlorine within a heavily polluted world these days. *Chlorine hasn't changed. Man's use of it has*.

It is becoming clear that chlorine is a chemical whose time has passed. We never dreamed that everyday chlorine could be so dangerous for human health because most of us have grown up with chlorine products. Decades ago our public water supplies were less polluted, and a few drops of chlorine could purify a lot of water. With all the pollution today, it's as if we are mixing

<u>dirty water with poisonous amounts of chlorine *hoping* it will stay clean.</u>

Here's a good example: chlorine at water treatment plants is unstable and easily separates from the water. This means the treatment plants have to add higher levels of chlorine so they can be sure some chlorine will remain in the water when it reaches your home. Because of chlorine's volatility, water systems have recently started treating tap water with chloramine instead of chlorine, and more water treatment plants seem to be switching to chloramine. Chloramine is a combination of chlorine and ammonia and is much more stable than chlorine. It won't dissolve from the water as easily, (leaving both chlorine and ammonia as by-products) and it isn't as likely to combine with other chemicals. But, chloramine isn't as good at killing microorganisms as chlorine, so higher levels of chloramine are often used in our water.

There is a major problem that can occur if your water is treated with chloramine: if you use a dechlorinator to protect a fish tank or an ornamental pond, or simply to dechlorinate your drinking water, the dechlorinator will eliminate the chlorine portion of the chloramines. Once the chlorine is eliminated, it leaves ammonia free within the water. So, if you use a simple dechlorinator, you are solving one problem (chlorine), but creating a new problem (ammonia).

Organochlorines are the combination of chlorine and organic substances. Pesticides, plastics, paints, dyes, deodorants, bleaching agents, refrigerants, wood preservers and cleaning solvents are common examples of products created by combining chlorine and petroleum. Organochlorines typically do not like water (hydrophobic) and are attracted to animal fats, including lipids (lipophilic), which is bad news for living creatures. Most organochlorines do not readily dissolve in water but instead gravitate toward fat-containing organisms where they "bioaccumulate" as they move up the food chain, from fish to man. Organochlorines in the tissues of some fish species, for example, have been measured 150 times greater than their level in the surrounding water. We humans are not exempt.

Dr. Jack Vallentyne, Senior Scientist, Canada Centre for Inland Waters, Burlington, Ontario stated: "Toxic chemicals, in large part organochlorines, have impaired and are impairing the natural populations of fish, reptiles, birds and mammals in the Great Lakes Basin. The concentrations of organochlorines in these wild populations are in the same general range as those found in human populations. Because of their short generation times, populations of fish and wildlife may be showing effects that will appear later in human populations. On this basis, and direct evidence from a limited number of human studies, the reports also concluded that there is a clear threat to human health. The dimensions of the human health threat are not well known."

Chlorine In Your Swimming Pool And In Your Diet Cola

Public pools are typically treated with chlorine-based disinfectants to help keep kids safe from the spread of infectious diseases while swimming. A study published in the June 2003 issue of *Occupational and Environmental Medicine* magazine demonstrated the downside of these chlorine products. The layer of chlorine gases hovering just above the water has the potential to damage your lungs and cause asthma. *The chlorine that stings your eyes can also "sting" the sensitive tissue of the lungs.* The risks are highest in indoor pools, and the lower the ceiling, the higher the risk.

In studying 1,881 children, researchers found a direct correlation between the total cumulative time a child spent splashing in an indoor pool with the risk that child developed asthma. They also found that blood levels of lung proteins rose immediately after swimming because the protective membranes in the lungs became temporarily open passages.

In most countries, certain pool chemicals have to be registered with their Department of Agricultures due to the volatility and toxicity of the chlorine-containing ingredients. The chlorine base of most commercial swimming pool treatments is added to the pool daily or every other day to control bacteria in the water. Algae in swimming pools, nevertheless, require a different arsenal of chemicals, and their chemical labels make for some heavy reading. These products are harming birds and killing honeybees that drink from pool water containing chloride compounds. (See the end of this chapter for alternative ways to keep your pool naturally clean.)

"If all the swimming pools used the same products," writes Dr. John Ledger in his article *The Environmental Impact of Swimming Pools*, "theoretically 650 million bees would be killed every week in the summer time."

Beware of breathing the chlorine fumes from tap water, hot tubs, swimming pools, and cleaning products. Not only can these chlorine vapors irritate your lungs, but they can pose a serious risk to people suffering from asthma, emphysema, and chronic heart conditions. Poorly ventilated areas increase this exposure. Many household products containing chlorine can be absorbed through the skin. Read your labels – many chorine-free cleansers are on the market now.

Asthma Alert
I recommend that people with asthma and other breathing conditions, especially young children, DO NOT use Splenda products containing sucralose or aspartame (generic or in NutraSweet/Equal). If you are currently using products containing these chemicals and are experiencing increased breathing difficulties, stop use immediately to determine if it is having an adverse effect on your breathing.

More Side Effects Of Chlorine—Birth Defects, Stillbirths, Cancer and Death

I have ornamental ponds in my yard with large Koi fish. I use a chemical de-chlorinator when I refill the ponds with tap water during the hot summer months. Any pond or aquarium owner knows that typically you do not need to add the extra chemicals (from a de-chlorinator) if you are merely "topping" off your pond - or you *shouldn't* need to, that is. The pond owners' "rule-of-thumb": when adding one-third or less of tap water to fill your pond, no chemical de-chlorinator needs to be added. But one dry Texas afternoon, I added a relatively small amount of water to my largest pond (an 800-gallon pond). Within an hour, all of my fifteen-inch Koi were dead, and the smell of chlorine vapors was evidence as to what killed my four year-old fish.

Chlorine apparently doesn't agree with living creatures. Doesn't this say something about fish or humans ingesting this chemical?

> **Do You Drink Eight Glasses Of Chlorine Per Day?**
> Would you drink a cup of pesticides? What about a cup
> of chemical water? As with the animal kingdom, so it is
> with human beings, especially fetuses and small children.
> Chlorine can make a human sick very quickly, and can
> destroy the good bacteria that keep the intestinal tract
> healthy.

Researchers Agree

According to recent research in Europe, pregnant women in
their first trimester who drink five or more glasses of chlorinated
tap water a day may be at a much higher risk of miscarriage than
women who drink non-chlorinated water.

A Norwegian study of 141,000 births over a three-year period
found a fourteen percent increased risk of birth defects in
areas with chlorinated water. Scientists have already found an
association between chlorine and an increased risk of bowel,
kidney and bladder cancer, but this is the first time a link has
been verified with higher levels of spina bifida.

Norwegian research scientist Dr. Per Magnus states, "We know
there are chemicals released by the action of chlorine. We have
observed mutations found in babies. We are in a unique position
in Norway to make these observations because in some areas, our
water comes from the mountains and doesn't require cleaning
with chlorine."

His statement is alarming. The chlorinated areas show
evidence of cancer. The unchlorinated areas do not. Splenda
manufacturers say the chlorine in their sweetener will pass
harmlessly out of your body. What if it doesn't? Chlorine is a
dangerous carcinogen according to the research. Do you really

want it inside *your* body? Keep in mind that we continue to use popular manmade pharmaceuticals such as Vioxx®, which was FDA-approved, yet abruptly pulled off the market. <u>Think ahead!</u> These companies may not have all the data in until it's too late for the consumer.

Concerned that chlorine in drinking water may cause spina bifida and stillbirths, the British government has ordered an independent study on chlorine-treated drinking water. Scientists from Imperial College, London University, are interested in the research from doctors in Norway, Canada and the United States reporting higher levels of birth defects in areas where chlorine is used, as compared with areas where drinking water is treated by alternative methods.

John Fawell, a leading specialist on water quality and an independent industry consultant, says, "The people who have done this work in Norway and in the United States are reputable researchers, and now water companies have commissioned their own research from London University." All of Britain's and the United States' water companies chlorinate their public water supplies. The only people who use non-chlorinated water are those with their own water wells.

A strong link was found in ten of the eleven studies that examined the link between chlorinated drinking water and bladder cancer. One study in Ontario, conducted with funding from Health Canada, found fourteen percent to sixteen percent of bladder cancers in Ontario showed a direct correlation to drinking water containing high levels of chlorine byproducts. At Dalhousie University, Nova Scotia, Canada, researchers found that high levels of trihalomethanes, a byproduct of chlorine in drinking water, significantly increased the risk of stillbirth.

But McNeil Nutritionals, the manufacturer of Splenda, still maintains sucralose is safe to consume. G.D. Searle, the manufacturer of NutraSweet, has maintained over the past 20 years that the methanol in aspartame is safe to consume. Now look at the tremendous amount of evidence proving aspartame is not safe. Let's learn from our past mistakes and not repeat the same patterns with sucralose.

Chlorine Used As A Weapon

During World War I, chlorine and mustard gas (made from chlorine called phosgene) were used against enemy soldiers as chemical weapons. During World War II, both opposing sides worked diligently to invent poisonous weapons far more destructive than mustard gas. As Rachel Carson explained in 1962 in her book Silent Spring, "WWII marked the rapid acceleration of experiments to combine gaseous chlorine with organic matter by combining carbon and hydrogen atoms, the building blocks of all life on earth. Many of these substances were tried out on insects, and when the war ended, they were unleashed on agricultural pests. DDT is one notable 'creation' of Second World War laboratories."

The chemical industry mushroomed in the 1950s, and at the forefront were chlorine combined with carbon (chlorocarbons) and chlorine/petroleum mixtures.

According to records on file with the Environmental Agency's Toxic Release Inventory (TRI) database, McNeil's McIntosh, Alabama plant (where Splenda is manufactured in the United States) released undetermined amounts of phosgene into the environment in 2000-2002.

TruthAboutSplenda.com writes about the following patent filed in the US Patent Office for production of sucralose:

One paragraph of this patent reads:
"On a laboratory scale, the crude chlorination product may be quenched in a batch operation by the addition (in one portion) of one molar equivalent (basis *phosgene*) of ice-cold aqueous solutions or slurries of the alkali or alkaline earth metal hydroxides. In one embodiment, the alkaline agents may include the hydroxides of sodium, potassium, and calcium. In a specific embodiment, more dilute aqueous alkaline solutions, such as about 3 to 4N sodium hydroxide, may be used. Broader ranges of concentration may also be used such as, about 2 to about 8N sodium hydroxide. At lower concentrations, precipitation of salts is reduced or avoided, which significantly reduces the amount of solids the process stream can accommodate. However, when the concentration becomes too low (e.g., below about 2N), the product stream may become diluted to an extent that may adversely affect the efficiency of the process. [0036]"

Phosgene Oxime is a chemical warfare agent. It is also very corrosive to most metals and is a high priority risk for HAZMAT engineers (Hazardous Waste and Emergency Responders). This chemical should not be allowed public access, nor, in my professional opinion, should it be permitted access by a general manufacturing lab.

As a HAZMAT engineer, I can tell you that there are similarities between symptoms due to phosgene exposure and current reported reactions to Splenda. (See Case Histories, Chapter Seven.)

Direct phosgene exposure mocks chlorine exposure with burning of the lungs, eyes, nose, and skin. It will also burn the internal organs if swallowed, but do not induce vomiting – treat with milk and charcoal and encourage diarrhea rather than vomiting.

Phosgene Oxime is nasty – like anthrax nasty.

Since phosgene is used selectively in the manufacture of isocyanates, polycarbonates and acid chlorides (mostly in pesticides and defoliators for public and military use), it drives the point home for our concern about abundant use of chlorine in our society today. (It is in over 60,000 products.) This is alarming, considering the volatility of chlorine and its ability to readily combine with other molecules, as in DDT.

Progressing from "merely dangerous" to "extremely dangerous" are the dioxins and the organochlorines in the group of chlorine chemicals known as Persistent Organic Pollutants (POPs). "They threaten the health and well-being of humans and wildlife in every region of the world," says John Buccini, a Canadian government representative to the United Nations Environmental Program (UNEP).

In study after study, exposure to these chemicals has demonstrated an increase in the risk of cancer and birth defects among wildlife. They provoke allergic reactions and damage the nervous, reproductive and immune systems of animals. Some dioxins and organochlorines mimic the hormone estrogen (called xenoestrogens), thus altering wildlife in ways that diminish their "ability and interest" in producing offspring. Some researchers believe these chemicals are related to the recent decrease in human sperm counts. Until recently, the presence of these ever-present chemicals raised little concern among scientists and government regulators because their concentration in humans and in the environment once appeared to be low. But a growing group of researchers and scientists are now considering the notion that these chemicals—found in everything from pesticides to plastics—may be causing problems in human beings. Scientists are now starting to use the term "signal disruptions" when talking about environmental hormones and refer to the concept of environmental hormones as "the endocrine hypothesis."

Dioxins and organochlorines are also some of the most enduring chlorine compounds. Once introduced into the environment it can take years, even decades, for POPs to break down to less damaging forms. As if this was not reason enough to be cautious, POPs have one final fatal flaw— **they are soluble in your fat and tend to remain in your body for long periods of time**. Your fatty tissues absorb POPs like a sponge draws water. UNEP scientists state that in some animals, POPs have been detected at levels 70,000 times higher than in their surroundings. DDT is a good example of a POP.

Splenda and DDT

According to Consumers Research Magazine, concern has been raised about sucralose being a chlorinated molecule because chlorinated molecules were used in the now-banned pesticide DDT, which accumulates in animal body fat. (DDT is an organochloride insecticide.)

While writing this book, McNeil Nutritionals' Dr. Leslie Goldsmith sent me a letter that stated, "It is unscientific and misleading to compare sucralose to pesticides like DDT. The two items are very different in composition and behavior. Sucralose is non-toxic, poorly absorbed and does not accumulate in the body. DDT is highly toxic, soluble in fat and accumulates in the body. There is absolutely no need for concern about the safety of sucralose due to <u>the chlorine molecule used in its manufacture</u>."

But, Dr. Goldsmith, they both are chlorinated molecules. Does your body know the difference?

- A "chlorocarbon" is any chlorine-containing compound. *(This is what is in Splenda.)*
- A "chlorinated molecule" is a molecule that has chlorine in its chemical arrangement. *(This is what is in Splenda.)*
- A "chlorocarbohydrate" appears to be the "new term"

that McNeil Nutritionals has coined for the chemical compound containing chlorine and sucrose. *(This is Splenda.)*

It would seem that by creating a new chemical category, McNeil would hope to avoid many of the negative associations of the chlorine-containing compounds described above. "I have never heard of a chlorocarbohydrate," explains Kelly Goyen, CEO of Empirical Laboratories. "This is a non-standard term according to my references and to the chemists on my staff. According to orthodox chemistry, I would treat this compound as any chlorine-containing compound molecule that has chlorine in its chemical arrangement. I see nothing special about it."

A Global Chlorine Ban?

John Williamson says it best in his article *Chlorine Quandary*: "If civilization has a smell, it is the cleansing scent of chlorine bleach. Its barely detectable aroma announces the water is safe, the surroundings are sanitary ... It is a bully of a chemical that punches through the cell walls of bacteria and shatters viruses. Use chlorine to disinfect a water supply—or to deliver it. Chlorine is also a prime ingredient in making plastic pipes. Chlorine-based pesticides civilized the tropics by eradicating disease-carrying mosquitoes and timber-chomping termites. Chlorine-based refrigerants put safe refrigerators in our kitchens and air conditioning in our cars. You would be hard pressed to find any industry that could exist without at least one chlorine-containing chemical. And it is precisely because of this popularity that a growing number of environmental scientists and public health experts agree that *chlorine should be banned*."

In December 2000, diplomats from 122 countries met in Johannesburg, South Africa to take action against the extensive use and toxic effects of chlorine. With sufficient research results presented, the international consensus was that nature had endured enough damage. "This new treaty will protect present and future generations from the cancers, birth defects and other tragedies caused by Persistent Organic Pollutants (POPs)," said Dr. John Buccini, who chaired the session.

The treaty marked a dozen chlorine-containing compounds for banishment. Eight are pesticides:

- DDT is the most familiar, and the other pesticides are:
  1. Aldrin
  2. Chlordane
  3. Dieldrin
  4. Endrin
  5. Heptachlor
  6. Mirex
  7. Toxaphene

- Two are industrial chemicals:
  1. PCBs (used to line utility poles, as a paint additive, and in plastics)
  2. Hexachlorobenzene (used in the manufacturing of fireworks, ammunition, synthetic rubber and pesticides, and a byproduct of manufacturing carbon tetrachloride and similar cleaning compounds)

- Dioxins and furans (released in the environment from the making of pesticides, polyvinyl chloride and chlorinated solvents)

Sources Of Chlorine In Your Daily Life

Cancer-causing residue from chlorine bleaching can be found in products like coffee filters, chlorine-bleached paper, disposable diapers, paper towels and bathroom tissue. Dioxins (chlorine-containing compounds) are recognized as one of the most carcinogenic chemicals known to science and have been linked to:

1. Endometriosis
2. Immune system impairment
3. Diabetes
4. Neurotoxicity
5. Birth defects (including fetal death)
6. Decreased fertility
7. Testicular atrophy
8. Reproductive dysfunction in both women and men

Thanks to chlorine pollution, Americans are exposed to a daily amount of chlorine toxins 300 to 600 times greater than the EPA's "safe" dose. Monitoring chlorine-containing products from animal feed to artificial sweeteners is a critical step in reducing human exposure to chlorine because <u>ninety-five percent of exposure to chlorine compounds occurs through the diet,</u> according to the U.S. Environmental Protection Agency and the U.S. Department of Agriculture.

Industry Is Beginning To Change Its View Of Chlorine
Ben & Jerry's® ice cream has the following printed on their carton:

"This is an unbleached 'eco-pint.' Bleaching paper with chlorine releases different dioxins, one of which the EPA identifies as the most toxic ever created. This eco-pint is part of our efforts to use environmentally safe packaging. Enjoy!"

Way to go, B&J!

More Chlorine-Based Poisons

Along with common manufactured chlorine comes a long and dangerous list of pollutants:

- Chlorofluorocarbons (CFCs) were banned in North America in 1997 due to their destruction of the ozone layer. Scientists predict it will take seventy-five to one hundred years for the ozone layer to fully recover.

- Polychlorinated biphenyls (PCBs) were widely used as electrical insulators until they were banned in the 1970s. PCBs remaining in the environment continue to damage wildlife reproduction, cause birth defects, and suppress the immune system of all living creatures.

- The North American pulp and paper industry currently pump one hundred million tons of organochlorines—including dioxins and furans—into our waterways each year.

- Household chlorine bleach produces trace amounts of chloroform, a known animal carcinogen and suspected human carcinogen.

Most of the chemicals produced in the laboratory using chlorine and carbon are still <u>unknown to nature</u>. They resist breakdown and deposit (bioaccumulate) in both the environment and in animal body fat. Often chlorine and its breakdown byproducts are very slow to decompose, and, in some cases, it may take years or decades to completely break down. Some chlorine compounds actually become more toxic once unleashed in the environment.

> Today, deposition of chlorine <u>within the human body</u> is an increasing reality, and the chlorine compound we must now add to this list is <u>chlorinated sucrose</u>—the "newly-marketed chlorocarbohydrate" (chlorocarbon) found in food products with unknown side effects from long-term internal use.

What To Do If Exposed To Chlorine

According to the CDC's (Centers for Disease Control and Prevention), if you have been exposed to <u>manmade</u> chlorine, seek emergency medical care immediately. Do not induce vomiting. If chlorine is on the skin or in the eyes, flush with lots of water for at least fifteen minutes. If chlorine is swallowed, drink water immediately.

Symptoms of chlorine poisoning are:

A. Respiratory
1. Breathing difficulty (typically from inhalation)
2. Throat swelling (which may also cause breathing difficulty)

B. Eyes, Ears, Nose And Throat
1. Severe pain in the throat
2. Severe pain or burning in the nose, eyes, ears, lips or tongue
3. Loss of vision

C. Gastrointestinal
1. Severe abdominal pain
2. Vomiting
3. Burns of the esophagus (food pipe)
4. Vomiting blood
5. Blood in the stool

D. Heart And Blood Vessels
1. Hypotension (low blood pressure) develops rapidly
2. Collapse

E. Skin
1. Irritation
2. Burn
3. Necrosis (holes) in the skin or underlying tissues

F. Blood
1. Severe changes in pH (too much or too little acid in the blood, which leads to damage in all of the body organs)

Considering the severity of these side effects, do you really want to risk regularly exposing your child or loved ones to a product that contains this class of chemicals, and has not had an extensive enough history to confirm its safety?

Is Chlorine Ever "Good"?

Yes, but only when it occurs <u>naturally</u> in foods in *trace* amounts. These are what Leslie Goldsmith from McNeil referred to in melons, mushrooms, and tomatoes in Chapter One. But this is natural chlorine – not Splenda's manmade chlorine. With synthetic versions of chlorine, you must be cautious, as it is impossible to predict all potential complications on human health.

Chlorine found in minute amounts in <u>nature</u> helps your liver cleanse, while OSHA has warned us that <u>synthetic</u> forms of chlorine can burn your internal organs. For example, a tomato is a <u>natural</u> food source of chlorine, but it contains no *<u>manmade</u>* amounts of chlorine. A tomato contains many more minerals as well, and unlike Splenda, <u>its chlorine molecules have not been replaced with laboratory halogens, and no molecules have been removed to prevent the chlorine in the tomato from digesting (as in sucralose)</u>. Along with organic chlorine, a tomato contains:

1. Sulphur
2. Potassium and sodium in combination
3. Phosphorus
4. Silicon (good for the skin)
5. Lycopene (cancer prevention)

Edible mushrooms do not contain manmade chlorine because the chemical damages the network of their feathery mycelia, the "ribs" underneath the umbrellas. These mycelia, often seen when turning over compost, are what the mushroom uses to absorb food and maintain the required moisture to make it a "mushroom." Most growers supply a regular spray of "de-chlorinated" water on their yields to achieve the perfect moisture conditions for growing.

In her article "Low Cost Mushroom Production at Home," Arzeena Hamir writes, "Using the right water, however, is critical. Well water or rainwater is best, as it doesn't contain any manufactured chlorine. If none of these are available, leave a bucket of water to stand overnight to allow the chemical chlorine to evaporate."

Reducing Your Exposure To Chlorine

A healthy diet and lifestyle are the best ways to reduce exposure to chlorine. By avoiding, or at least decreasing your consumption of processed foods, you significantly reduce your chances of eating any manmade chlorine found in chlorinated water and pesticides sprayed on the crops. Combine this with clean, organic vegetables and naturally raised meat and eggs, you will be on the right health track.

The Chlorine Chemistry Council backs the efforts to better understand the role that chlorine plays in human health and the environment. Supporting their commitment to science education and to local communities, the CCC stated, "We are working to further reduce emissions into the food supply, while at the same time provide the building blocks of chlorine chemistry that help produce essential products that make our lives safer, healthier and more convenient."

Dr. John Marshall of the Pure Water Association, an American consumer group campaigning for safer drinking water, states, "It shows we should be paying more attention to the chemicals we put in our drinking water and should be looking for other alternatives to chlorination. A number of safe, non-toxic options exist, such as treating water with ozone gas or ultra violet light."

The Norwegian government has also ordered more research to be done. Concerned families have begun filtering their tap water with a popular method of placing sachets of coral sand dredged from Norwegian fjords into the water before it is consumed, removing all traces of chlorine after fifteen minutes.

Chlorine: In Your Swimming Pool And In Your Diet Cola

Here are some safety tips you can follow to reduce your daily chlorine exposure:

1. Filter your tap water in your kitchen, bath and shower or any other source that you will consume or expose your body to chlorinated water
2. Convert your chlorinated swimming pool to a salt water pool or a system that uses ozone or peroxide to clean the pool
3. Eat organic foods if at all possible
4. Use chlorine-free packaging
5. Switch to non-chlorine-based cleaning products
6. Avoid chlorine-bleached feminine products, disposable diapers and paper products like toilet paper and paper towels

And now,

7. *Consider avoiding deliberate consumption of artificial sweeteners containing chlorine!*

CHAPTER 3

Splenda Product List

As of May 2004 when I completed the first edition of this book, the list at the time was over 3,000 products containing Splenda, and was thirty-four pages in length. Today, the list has substantially lengthened, and now includes Diet Coke®, NutraSweet's exclusive for over twenty years.

I have briefly listed the major food categories in this chapter, and have included the complete file to download from my website www.splendaexposed.com. Note: some of these products are not labeled *sugar-free*, and some products may also be combined with *aspartame* and other chemical sugar substitutes. My best advice: read ALL the labels on anything you buy for your or your children's safety.

This list includes a variety of foods and food products, pharmaceuticals and children's medications, vitamin supplements, protein powders, protein bars, weight loss products, liquid and powdered drinks, popcorn, gums, mints, toothpaste, and water.

For detailed product information, reference my website http://www.splendaexposed.com.

List Of U.S. Products With Splenda Brand Sweetener

I. Carbonated Beverages

Dr. Pepper/Seven Up, Inc.
§ Diet Rite®
§ Diet RC® Cola

Urban Juice and Soda Co.
§ Jones Juice
§ Slim Jones™ Diet Soda

Jones Soda Co.
§ Jones Naturals

Roadside Beverage L.L.C.
§ Root 66 Diet Root Beer®

Clearly Canadian Beverages (U.S.) Corp.
§ Diet Clearly Canadian®

Briar's USA, Inc.
§ Briar's Diet

Stewart's Beverages, Inc.
§ S Diet

Kroger Company (Private Label)
§ Light Juice Cocktail
§ Crystal Clear Sugar Free Sparkling Water

7-Eleven Inc. (Private Label)
§ Classic Selection Sugar Free Sparkling Water

Splenda Product List

Family Dollar (Private Label)
§ Diet Cola

Adirondack Beverages
§ Waist Watcher Diet Carbonated Soft Drinks

White Rock Products Corporation
§ White Rock®

Napa Valley Beverage Company
§ Napa Valley Sparkling Beverages

Star Beverage Co.
§ Diet Reach for the Star

Boylan Bottling Company
§ Boylan's Diet

Upstate Beverages, Inc.
§ Upstate Diet Cola (fountain)

Monarch Beverage, Inc.
§ Monarch Diet Cola (fountain)

D'Best Dispensers
§ D'Best Diet Cola (fountain)

Rivella (USA) Inc.
§ Diet Rivella

A-Treat Bottling Co.
§ Diet A-Treat

National Beverage Co.
§ Cascadia Sparkling Water with Juice
§ Crystal Bay Sparkling Water

§ Diet Shasta

Dollar General
§ Clover Valley Soft Drink

Caroline Beverage Company
§ Cheerwine Diet

Labatt
§ Labatt Light Source

II. Gelatins, Puddings, And Fillings

Knouse Foods, Inc.
§ Lucky Leaf® Lite "No Sugar Added"
§ Musselman's® "Lite" Applesauce

ConAgra Grocery Products Company
§ Jolly Rancher Sugar Free Gel Snacks

III. Still Beverages

Ocean Spray Cranberries, Inc.
§ Ocean Spray® Light Juice Drinks
§ Ocean Spray® Lightstyle Juice Drinks

Nestlé USA
§ Nestlé Nescafé Frothé Coffee Drink
§ Nestlé Coffee-mate®

Snapple Beverage Corporation
§ Diet Snapple Iced Tea
§ Mistic Zero Calorie Diet Drink
§ Mistic Juice and Tea Beverages

Splenda Product List

J.M. Smucker Company
  § Smucker's Diet Beverage

Arizona Beverage Company
  § Arizona WaterAid
  § Arizona Diet Lemon Iced Tea
  § Arizona Diet Raspberry Iced Tea
  § Arizona Diet Peach Iced Tea
  § Arizona Diet Green Tea with Ginseng and Honey
  § Blue Luna Café™
  § Arizona Iced Coffee

American Quality Beverages
  § Z'Lektra Sport
  § AquaSport

Quaker
  § Propel Fitness Water

Veryfine Products, Inc.
  § Veryfine® Fruit2O™
  § Veryfine Fruit2O
  § Veryfine Fruit2O Plus
  § Veryfine Fruit2O Ice

Kraft Foods, Inc.
  § Crystal Light Ready-To-Drink

Talking Rain® Beverage Co., Inc.
  § Diet Ice Botanicals™

Swiss Natural Foods, Inc.
  § Swiss Natural

ChampionLyte, Inc.
  § ChampionLyte Sugar Free Sports Drink

Aloe Splash, Inc.
§ Aloe Splash

South Beach Beverages (SoBe)
§ SoBe Lean™ Sugar Free

Nantucket Allserve, Inc.
§ Squeezed Nectars™

Daily's Juice Products division of American Beverage Corp.
§ Diet Guzzler
§ Daily's®
§ Little Hug (Assorted Flavors)
§ Teeni (Assorted Flavors)
§ Fruit Stand (Assorted Flavors)
§ Hummy (Assorted Flavors)

Hansen's Natural Corporation
§ Hansen's Smoothie
§ Diet Hasen's
§ Hansen's Diet Energy Fuel
§ Hansen's Energy Water

Low Carb Living, Inc.
§ BaJa Bob's

Campbell Soup Supply Co.
§ Diet V8 Splash®

Vermont Pure
§ Vermont Pure Essence™ Spring Water

Clearly Canadian Beverage Company
§ Reebok Fitness Water

Langer Juice Company, Inc.
§ Langer's Diet Juice

Calypso Ice Beverages
§ Calypso Ice

Adirondack
§ Natural Spring Water

Damon Industries
§ Fruitful Diet Juice

Cott Beverages
§ A&P Master Choice Sparkling Water

Jel Sert
§ Mondo Fruit Squeezers

American Beverage Corporation
§ Juice Xplosion Fruit Drink

Mott's
§ Las Fuentes Aguas Frescas Light

IV. Sauces, Toppings, And Syrups

Aurora Foods, Inc.
§ Log Cabin® Sugar Free Low Calorie Syrup

Hain Food Group
§ Estee Smart Treats Sugar Free Syrup
§ Estee Sugar Free Wafers

R. Torre & Company
§ Torani Coffee Flavoring Syrups

DaVinci Gourmet®, Ltd.
§ DaVinci Gourmet Sugar Free Syrups
§ DaVinci Gourmet Sugar Free Spiced Chai
§ DaVinci Gourmet Sugar Free Lemon Tea

Hammer Corporation
§ Armands Flavored Syrups
§ Spray Candy

Maple Grove Farms
§ Cozy Cottage Sugar Free Syrup
§ Vermont Sugar Free Syrup

Walden Farms, Inc.
§ Walden Farms Calorie Free Salad Dressings

Nature's Flavors.com, Inc.
§ Nature's Flavors Syrups

Sorbee International Ltd.
§ Sorbee® Zero Sugar Syrup

Oscar Skollberg's Technique, subsidiary of Stearns and Lehman
§ Oscar's Light Syrup and Oscar's Sugar Free Syrups

Silos Inn
§ Ernie's Silos Inn "Low Sugar" BBQ Sauce

Carriage House Company
§ WalMart Great Value Sugar Free Chocolate Syrup

V. Processed Fruits

Dole Packaged Foods Company
§ Dole Fruit-N-Gel Bowls
§ Dole Reduced Sugar Fruit N' Gel Bowls

E.D. Smith
§ DeLightful Fruit Spreads

Del Monte Foods
§ Del Monte Fruit & Gel To-Go Lite

B&G Foods
§ Polaner Sugar Free Fruit Spreads

VI. Chewing Gum

Warner-Lambert Co.
§ Trident for Kids™ Sugarless Gum Berry Bubble Gum

Church & Dwight
§ Arm & Hammer Dental Care for Kids Bubble Gum
§ Arm & Hammer Advance Breath Care Gum

Wm. Wrigley Jr. Company
§ Orbit Chewing Gum
§ Juicy Fruit Gum
§ Bubble Jug
§ Eclipse Flash Strips

Hershey Foods Corporation
§ Ice Breakers Chewing Gum
§ Ice Breakers Unleashed Chewing Gum

Twinlab
§ Thermogenic Diet Gum
§ Ripped Fuel Gum

Oak Leaf Confections, Canada
§ Jolt Gum – Caffeine Energy gum

Adams
§ Dentyne Fire Chewing Gum

Kraft
§ Altoids Strips

VII. Powdered Beverage Mixes

ConAgra Grocery Products Company
§ Swiss Miss® "No Sugar Added" Hot Cocoa Mix
§ Swiss Miss® "Fat Free" Hot Cocoa Mix Swiss Miss® Fat Free
§ Marshmallow Lovers Hot Cocoa Mix
§ Swiss Miss® Fat Free French Vanilla Hot Cocoa Mix
§ Swiss Miss® Diet Hot Cocoa Mix

4C Foods
§ 4C Light Iced Tea Mix

Nestle
§ Nescafe Iced Java

VIII. Nutritional Products

Worldwide Sport Nutrition
§ Pure Protein™ Meal Replacement bar
§ Pure Protein™ Shake

Atkins Nutritionals, Inc.
§ Atkins Advantage Bar™
§ Atkins Breakfast Bar
§ Atkins Endulge Bar
§ Atkins Shake Mix
§ Atkins Ready-to-Drink Shakes
§ Atkins Syrups
§ Atkins Muffin Mix

Nature's Best
§ VHT Totally Ripped Dietary Supplement
§ VHT Extreme Smoothie
§ Perfect Zero Carb Isopure™ Protein Mix
§ Perfect Low Carb Isopure™
§ Perfect Zero Carb Isopure Drink
§ Nature's Best Isopure Sport (various flavors)
§ Nature's Best Lemon Aide

Met-Rx® USA Inc., Anabolic Drive Series
§ After FX Meal Supplement
§ Protein Plus High Protein Food Bar
§ After FX Protein Food Bar (various flavors)
§ Glycemet
§ Met-Rx White Packet

MuscleLink™
§ Pro Fusion™

Unico Holdings, Inc.
§ Naturalyte Oral Electrolyte Solution

PTS Labs
§ Revital Squeezers® Oral Electrolyte Solution

Bionutritional Research Group
§ ProtoWhey Protein Drink Mix

Bioplex Nutrition
§ Simply Whites
§ Whey Plex 100% Whey Protein

California Engineered Foods
§ California Protein

Chemi-Source, Inc
§ Metabolic Response Modifiers CreActiv

Davedraper.com
§ Bomber Blend Protein Powder

Life Services Supplements
§ Keto

Maximum Human Performance
§ TRAC® Powder Supplement

Optim Nutrition
§ Optimum Muscle Defense

TKE, Inc.
§ TKE

SportPharma
§ Extra Protein Bars
§ Just Whey Protein Powder
§ Promax Protein Powder

Experimental Applied Sciences, Inc.
§ EAS Ribforce HP Effervescent Creative
§ EAS AdvantEdge Carb Control Ready-to-Drink Shake
§ EAS Myoplex Ready-to-Drink Shake
§ StrawberryEAS Myoplex Carb Sense Ready-to-Drink Shake

- § EAS AdvantEdge Carb Control Bars
- § EAS Myoplex Low Carb Bars
- § EAS Beta Blast – 2 varieties – with and without ephedra
- § EAS Results for Women Ready-to-Drink with Fewer Carbs
- § EAS Results for Women Carbonated Energy Drink (8.4oz)
- § EAS Results for Women Bars with Fewer Carbs
- § EAS AdvE HP Energy
- § EAS Cytovol
- § EAS Precision Protein
- § EAS Results for Women Thermogenic Drinks
- § EAS Myoplex Powder
- § EAS Myoplex Deluxe Powder

Nutrition for Life
- § Slender Age
- § M2 Power-Play

Rexall Sundown
- § TruSoy Protein Shakes
- § TruSoy Bars
- § Carb Solutions Bars
- § Carb Solutions Ready-to-Drink
- § Osteo Bi-Flex Fruit Chews
- § Sundown Pokemon Vitamins
- § Sundown Soy Protein Shake Powder
- § Protein Revolution Low Carb Bars
- § Protein Revolution Shake Mix

Ross Products
- § Pedialyte Oral Electrolyte Solution
- § Pedialyte Pops
- § Met-Rx Total Nutrition Powder

Twin Lab
- § Fuel Plex
- § Fuel Plex Lite

§ Metabolift High Protein, Low Carb Meal Replacement
§ Ripped Fuel Thermogenic Gum
§ Energy Fuel
§ XE RTD
§ XA RTD

Labrada Bodybuilding Nutrition
§ Low Carb Lean Body Protein Shake Mix
§ Lean Body Bars (variety of flavors)
§ Lean Body for Her Bars (variety of flavors)

Biochem
§ Ultimate Lo Carb Shake
§ Ultimate Lo Carb Smoothie
§ American Body Building

Cytodyne Technologies, Inc.
§ Methoxy – Pro Protein Drink Mix
§ Cytoplex Meal Replacement

Pinnacle Products
§ Bodyonics Androstat – 100 Poppers

Pacific Health Labs
§ Satietrol Appetite Control Beverage

Great Earth Great Body
§ MyoTechRx Protein Shake
§ Whey Excess
§ Creatine Explode

Natrol/ProLab
§ Lean Mass Pro35 Protein Drink
§ Metabolic Thyrolean Soy Protein Drink
§ Lean Mass Meal Replacement
§ Cory Everson's Solutions Soy Protein Shake

Splenda Product List

Beverly International Nutrition
- § Ultra Size (Protein Drink)
- § Muscle Provider Drink Mix
- § Port-A-Meal Muscle Provider

Advocare International
- § Heart Source Bar
- § POS H Rehydration Powder
- § Advocare® Turbo Shake
- § Advocare® Spark
- § Advocare® Sugar Free Spark

Fitness Labs Nutrition
- § Fitness Labs Whey Protein 80
- § Fitness Labs Whey Protein 90

Nutra Force, Inc.
- § Nutra Force Vitamin & Mineral Water

CytoSport, Inc.
- § Cytomax™ Exercise and Recovery Drink
- § Cytosport Muscle Milk

Wellness Lifestyles Inc.
- § American Longevity Nature's Whey

Omnitrition, Inc.
- § Pro Builder Protein Powder

Scientific Solution
- § Sugar Free EZ Memory
- § Sugar Free EZ Energy

Weight Perfect, Inc
- § Weight Perfect® High Soy

Amway Corporate
§ Nutrilite Triple Guard Echinacea Spray
§ Trim Advantage Meal Replacement Drink Mix
§ Trim Advantage Protein Bar

Nutrition Technologies Inc.
§ Glutapro Glutamine Enhanced Whey Protein

Wellness International
§ Pro-xtreme Protein Drink Mix

American Longevity
§ Nature's Whey™

Amerifit, Inc.
§ Sugar Free Glucosamine and Chondroitin
§ Sugar Free Sooth Herbs

Amerifit Nutrition, Inc.
§ Vitaball™ Vitamin Gumball

Biosport Inc.
§ Biosport

GNC
§ Mega Creatine
§ Mega MRP
§ Scan Diet Bars
§ Distance Drink
§ Mega Whey
§ Natural Brand Soy Protein

Splenda Product List

Optimum Nutrition
§ Opti-Soy Soy Protein
§ Complete Protein Diet Shake Mix
§ Complete Protein Diet Bars
§ ProComplex Protein Shake Mix

Muscletech Research and Development
§ Muscletech Nitro-Tech Ready-To-Drink Nutrition
§ Muscletech Nitro-Tech Ready-To-Drink Shake
§ Mesotech Nutrition Bar

Next Proteins International
§ Designer Whey Protein Powder
§ Designer Whey GlycerLean
§ Designer Whey Protein Blast Punch
§ Designer Whey Protein Bars

Advanced Metabolic, Inc.
§ Pentabasol Supplement Powder

Max Muscle, Inc.
§ Max Muscle® Protein Powder

Morinda Inc.
§ Tahitian Noni Tahiti Trim™ Complete Shake

Pure De-Lite Inc.
§ Pure De-Lite High Protein Low Carb Cookie

Baxter Healthcare Corporation
§ Pulse Women's Health Formula

Ketogenics, Inc.
§ Ketogenics™ Sugar Free Chocolate Crisp

Physician's Laboratories
§ Revival Soy Protein Drink Mixes
§ Revival Soy Low-Carb Protein Bars

Arizona Beverage Corporation
§ Arizona RTD Rx Total Trim

NuVim
§ NuVim RTD Be Healthy & Energetic Beverage

IX. Baked Goods

Heavenly Cheesecakes, Inc.
§ Heavenly Cheesecakes

Wilson's Foods, Inc.
§ Wilson's Fantastic Mini Wafers

Nabisco Biscuit Company, Division of Nabisco, Inc.
§ SnackWell's Sugar Free Sandwich Cookies

Sorbee International Ltd.
§ Sorbee® Sugar Free Cookies

Perestroika Products
§ Red Square

X. Specialty Products

Smokey Mountain Chew, Inc.
§ Smokey Mountain Snuff (non-tobacco)

ConAgra Foods Retail Products Company
§ Act II Popcorn

§ Orville Redenbacher's™ Gourmet Popping Corn

Jel Sert Company
§ Fla-Vor-Ice Lite
§ Sugar Free Pop-Ice

General Mills
§ Pop Secret Popcorn

Ramsey Popcorn Company, Inc.
§ Cousin Willie's Kettle Corn Microwave Popcorn

Weaver Popcorn
§ Pop Weaver Microwave Kettle Corn

American Popcorn Company
§ Jolly Time KettleMania
§ Jolly Time Healthy Pop Kettlecorn

Cannon Unlimited Inc.
§ Cannon's Sweet Chile

Blistex, Inc.
§ Herbal Answer Lip Protection

Church & Dwight Company, Inc.
§ Arm & Hammer Advance White Sensitive Formula
 Toothpaste
§ Arm & Hammer Advance Breath Care Mints

Kraft Foods, Inc.
§ Altoid Strips
§ Crystal Light Slurpees
§ It's Pasta Anytime Three Cheese Rotini

Life Services Supplements
§ Keto

Atkins Nutritionals
§ Weetabix Atkins Flakes

Jamieson Laboratories
§ Pro Medis

XI. Dairy Products

Well's Dairy Inc.
§ Blue Bunny Lite 85 yogurt
§ Blue Bunny No Sugar Added Reduced Fat Ice Cream
§ Blue Bunny No Sugar Added Fat Free Ice Cream
§ Blue Bunny Frozen Novelties
§ Blue Bunny Lite Chocolate Fat Free Milk

Velvet Ice Cream Company
§ Velvet "No Sugar Added" Ice Cream

Whitey's Ice Cream
§ Whitey's No Sugar Added Ice Cream (Various flavors)

Good Humor - Breyers Ice Cream
§ Breyers™ No Sugar Added Fruit Bars

Mister Cookie Face, Inc.
§ Mister Cookie Face No Sugar Added Vanilla Ice Cream
Sandwich
§ Mister Cookie Face No Sugar Added Vanilla Chocolate Ice
Cream Sandwich

Pierre's French Ice Cream Company
§ Pierre's® Slender™ No Sugar Added Reduced Fat Free Ice

Cream

H.P. Hood Inc.
§ Hood Fat Free Egg Nog

Anderson Erickson
§ YoLite Nonfat Yogurt

Southwest Foods, division of Brookshire Grocery Company
§ Goldenbrook® Farms LeCarb Frozen Dessert

Pecan Deluxe Candy Company
§ Various flavors & varieties of No Sugar Added inclusions & ribbons for ice cream

Kroger
§ No Sugar Added Ice Cream

Bravo Foods International
§ Slim Slammers No Sugar Added Milk

Dannon
§ Dannon Light 'n Fit Smoothie

Ultima Foods
§ Yoplait Source Yogurt

Cool Brands
§ Weight Watchers Smart Ones "No Sugar Added" Ice ream

XII. Confectionery Products

Goelitz Confectionery Co.
§ Sugar Free Tummy Bears
§ Sugar Free Jelly Belly (Jellybeans)

Sorbee® International Ltd.
§ Sorbee Lites Hard Candy

Shuster Marketing Corporation
§ Blitz Power Mints

Simply Lite Foods Corp.
§ Wafer Bars

Pavalor Advanced Technologies
§ Extreme Candy Spray

Hillside Candy Company
§ Go Lightly Hard Candy (Assorted Flavors)

Wal-Mart, Inc (Private Label)
§ Sugar Free Hard Candy (Assorted Flavors)

Estee, Inc.
§ Hard Candy (Assorted Flavors)

BestSweet Inc.
§ Baskin Robbins Sugar Free Smooth and Creamy Hard
  Candy

Wm. Wrigley Jr. Company
§ Thin Ice Strips

Nabisco
§ Lifesavers Minis

Hershey Foods
§ Hershey's Sugar Free Chocolate Candy
§ Reese's Sugar Free Chocolate Candy

XIII. Over The Counter RX

Whitehall Robbins
§ Robitussin Flu

NewAys International Oral Care
§ Toothpastes

Jamieson Laboratories
§ Jamieson Chewable C
§ Zinc Lozenges
§ Mega Kids Chewable Solotron Arthur with Iron

List Of Canadian Products With Splenda® Brand Sweetener

I. Still Beverages

A. Lassonde
§ Fruite Light
§ Rougemont Light
§ Tetley Lemon Diet Iced Tea

Loblaw Companies Limited
§ President's Choice
§ No Name Light Peach Drink

Leading Brands
§ Trek Fitness Water

McCain
§ McCain Light Lemon Iced Tea Frozen Concentrate

Neilson Dairy
§ California

Oshawa Group
§ Our Complements

Pride Beverages Ltd.
§ Pride of BC Diet
§ Diamond Grove

Ice Down Beverages
§ Ice Down Iced Coffee

Western Family
§ Western Family Light Cocktail

Shoppers Drug Mart
§ Life Brand Naturals Diet Lemon Iced Tea

Allen's Food Industries
§ Allen's Diet Lemon Iced Tea

A&P
§ Master's Choice

Jaffasweet Juices
§ Jaffa Squeeze Frozen Lemonade Concentrate
§ Equality Frozen Lemonade Concentrate

Nestle Canada
§ Nestle Iced Cappuccino Syrup

II. Carbonated Beverages

Cadbury Beverages Canada Inc.
§ Diet Crush

Davco Inc.
§ Diet Up John Cola Concentrate

Embouteillage Elite's
§ Diet Marque 1-2-3-4

Flavour Essence Products Inc.
§ Mystic Diet Beverage Mix

Beverages Kiri
§ Crème Soda with 50% less sugar
§ Strawberry with 50% less sugar
§ Lemon Lime with 50% less sugar
§ Ginger Ale with 50% less sugar
§ Orange with 50% less sugar

Seaman's Beverages Limited
§ Seaman's Diet Orange Pop

III. Chewing Gum And Confectionery

Kerr Bros
§ Light Mint Candies
§ Light Toffee
§ Light Sour Lemon
§ Light Fruit
§ Light Lollipops
§ Light Scotch Minis

Rito Mints
§ Rito Light Mints

Wrigley
§ Extra Sugar Free Gum

Adam's Brands
§ Trident Sugarless Gum
§ Dentyne Gum

IV. Baked Goods

Boulangerie Beausejour
§ Beausejour Light Pie

Champion Food Company
§ Champion No Sugar Added Wild Blueberry Pie

Lentia Enterprise
§ Dia-Bella Sponge Cake Mix
§ Dia-Bella Mousse Mix
§ Dia-Bella Fond Mix

Paradise Bakery
§ Reduced Calorie Cookies
§ Reduced Calorie Custard
§ Reduced Calorie Brownies

Valley Bakery
§ Valley Bakery Diabetic Carrot Muffins

V. Condiments And Sauces

Loblaw Companies Limited
- § President's Choice TGTBT
- § Memories

E.D. Smith
- § E.D. Smith Spread
- § E.D. Smith Sugar Free Syrup

J.M. Smuckers Canada
- § Smuckers Sugar Free Fruit Spread

Oscar Skollberg's Technique, subsidiary of Stearns and Lehman
- § Oscar's Light Syrup and Oscar's Sugar Free Syrups

VI. Frozen Foods

Kisko Products
- § Kisko Kids No Sugar Added Freeze Pops

Hershey Cabada
- § Mr. Freeze No Sugar Added Freeze Pops

Chapman's Ice Cream
- § Chapman's No Sugar Added Ice Cream

Oshawa Group
- § Smart Choice NO Sugar Added Freeze Pops

Western Family
- § Western Family No Sugar Added Freeze Pops

VII. Processed Fruit And Vegetable Products

CA Fruit Ltd.
§ CA Fruit Deluxe Chilled Fruit Salad

Leachy Orchards
§ Applesnax Apple Sauce

VIII. Yogurt

Yoplait
§ Source Yogurt

IX. Nutritionals

Interactive Nutrition
§ Interactive Nutrition Whey Wildberry

Champions Choice Advanced Nutrition
§ Creatine Citrate Lemonade

Confab
§ Vitamin C Supplement

Pro-Amino International Inc.
§ Pro-Amino Concentrate Drink

Future Nutrition
§ Prowhey
§ Meal RX
§ Absolute Power
§ Power Mass

Pulse Nutrition Solutions Inc.
§ Pulse

X. Pharmaceuticals And Otc

Warner-Lambert
§ Benylin First Defence

And the list is growing in number, day by day...

CHAPTER 4

Healthy Alternatives

Weight loss without sacrificing sweetness represents an enormous growth opportunity for the food and beverage industry worldwide. But as everyone knows, <u>the average human prefers taste to nutrition</u>. Let's see how we can reverse this trend.

The two safest choices to date are saccharin and stevia. Saccharin is actually similar to stevia in its origin. It originally came from a plant imported from China, and in its original form is a complex sugar extract from the plant itself. Stevia is extracted from a plant grown in South America and is also a complex sugar extract. In the beginning, saccharin was sold in tiny pin-sized pellets, and merely two or three were enough to add sweetness to coffee or iced tea. This is what I consider a natural sucrose (sugar) substitute.

Both stevia and saccharin (in their original forms) are complex plant carbohydrates, so they do not pass into the bloodstream, yet still deliver a natural sweetness. People complain that both can be bitter, but that is an easy problem to fix. <u>Don't use too much</u>. It's the same as seasoning a tomato with too much salt or pepper, or using too much garlic or oregano on lasagna. Start off slowly and add as you "taste test." Modern consumers are in the habit of using huge amounts of sugar, and they automatically *pour on* the equivalent of saccharin or stevia they would use for refined sugar or artificial sweeteners. If you simply use one-quarter the amount of saccharin or stevia for one serving of sugar, then the taste is pleasant, natural and not bitter.

The Straight Skinny On Saccharin

> ### NO, SACCHARIN DOES NOT CAUSE CANCER!
> Research proves it's safe. Read on!

THE SECRET TO SACCHARIN AND STEVIA: DON'T USE TOO MUCH OR THEY WILL TASTE BITTER.

I know I am starting this chapter on "healthy sweeteners" with an "artificial sweetener" most people think causes cancer, but saccharin is the safest of the "traditional" artificial choices and is actually one of the safest alternative sweeteners to use (if you insist on tearing open a colored packet, that is). Natural sugars such as Sucanat® and stevia are preferable over saccharin of course, but saccharin has less harmful side effects than the more modern artificial sweeteners (especially for the diabetic) and is readily available.

I consider the *original* saccharin a natural alternative, not a chemical one. Advertisers have painted a very different picture of saccharin over the past twenty years, though, and the politics behind "sodium saccharide" has left it with a bum rap.

Saccharin is actually a natural plant sugar derivative, and back in the day when saccharin was "accidentally" discovered, it was considered an authentic sugar substitute because it *was* the only known alternative to traditional sugar.

Unfortunately, today saccharin's molecules have been reproduced in the laboratory and the pink packet is filled with anti-caking agents and emulsifiers. Saccharin is no longer sourced to its origin, but is still the most natural choice of the "colorful paper packets." (Choose the pink packets—even if they have different brand names.)

The history of saccharin tells the story of its safety. In 1879, Constantine Fahlberg discovered the sweetness of saccharin by accident. While working on plant studies in the lab, he spilled some chemicals on his hand. Later while eating dinner, he noticed more sweetness on his bread. He traced the sweetness back to the spilled chemical, which he later named saccharin—a spin-off of saccharide (complex sugar).

By 1907, saccharin was used as a replacement for sugar in foods for diabetics. Since pure saccharin is not metabolized into the bloodstream, it is classified as a noncaloric sweetener. By the 1960s, it was used on a wider scale in the "diet" soft drink industry in Coca Cola's Tab® and Fresca®, but primarily due to the times, the diet industry never took off.

Saccharin was widely used in Europe during World War II because of a sugar shortage. My father starting using saccharin during World War II while stationed in India, and safely used it his entire lifetime. Most European countries used saccharin as their number one alternative sweetener of choice until NutraSweet lost its patent in the 1990s, spawning the introduction of many new chemical sweetener choices.

Why Was Saccharin Labeled As A Carcinogen In The 1960s? It appears saccharin was sacrificed to make room in the market for a new more profitable sweetener, NutraSweet/Equal.

In 1902, Monsanto Chemical Company gained its reputation by manufacturing **saccharin**, the company's first product. From

1903 through 1905, their entire saccharin output was shipped to the growing new soft drink company in Georgia named **The Coca-Cola Company**®.

According to Monsanto's company history, the U.S. government filed suit over the safety of saccharin *at Monsanto's request* in 1917. Monsanto used the suit as a test case for safety, and the suit was dismissed in 1925. This gave saccharin much-needed government approval for safety early on.

Then, curiously, in 1969 saccharin was suddenly questioned as a carcinogen—out of the blue. No reputable scientific proof was ever presented. <u>Note: this was the year NutraSweet applied for their first patent.</u>

Something most people never realized is the toxicity study was actually done using a blend of cyclamate and saccharin, and the results were "interpreted" as linking <u>cyclamate</u>—not saccharin—to bladder cancer in rats. Researchers fed laboratory mice sweetened water that was equivalent to 800 cans of saccharin/cyclamate every day from birth until death. In this <u>one</u> test, <u>one</u> mouse developed bladder cancer, and the results were submitted to the FDA requesting a cancer warning be placed on all saccharin products. Cyclamate was banned in 1970. No further testing was performed. And why didn't the manufacturer of saccharin fight back? Read on...

Eight years after the "saccharin/cancer" scare, G.D. Searle & Co. (the original NutraSweet manufacturer) finally secured FDA approval for NutraSweet. It prepared to purchase Monsanto, the original saccharin manufacturer. Soon, NutraSweet and saccharin (its only competitor) were owned by the same company—Monsanto Chemical. <u>The FDA finally (at this time) printed cancer warnings on saccharin packets the year NutraSweet came onto the market</u>. So, saccharin's manufacturer didn't fight back because both saccharin and aspartame were now owned and marketed by the same company- Monsanto.

<u>Monsanto sold The NutraSweet Company in 2000. In 2001, the cancer warning was removed from saccharin products.</u> Saccharin is now deemed safe for human consumption—*once again.*

After more than one hundred years of use worldwide, there have only been six complaints against saccharin registered with the FDA. Yet, saccharin is the most questioned food ingredient among the chemical sweeteners—the only sweetener labeled as a possible carcinogen. <u>Extensive research on human populations has established no association between saccharin and cancer.</u> In fact, more than thirty human studies have been performed and all support saccharin's safety at human levels of consumption. It appears the corporate saccharin cancer studies in the late 1960s were indeed questionable and an example of marketing genius to promote a new sweetener product.

Cumberland Packing Corp., Brooklyn, New York, has manufactured Sweet'N Low® containing saccharin for over forty years. In 2002, over twenty years after the flawed cancer studies, Cumberland hailed the U.S. Congress for honoring the original moratorium agreement (made back in 1981) to lift the cancer warning and grant saccharin a clean bill of health.

"We were finally able to remove the cancer warning from all of our products, and that was a big deal," Cumberland marketing director says. "We went so far as to replace the cancer warning with the Good Housekeeping Seal. We turned unfair negatives into an immediate positive."

(See Appendix VII for the FDA Report on Saccharin Safety.)

Saccharin—The Oldest Artificial Sweetener

If it were still processed from a natural source, saccharin could be considered a natural sugar like stevia and Sucanat. But after World War II, saccharin fell prey to laboratory manufacturing. It is now processed using manmade components to curb manufacturing costs, but for the most part saccharin's chemical make-up is simple—especially in comparison to the manufacturing process of the other chemical sweeteners, such as sucralose (made with chlorine) and aspartame (made with methanol).

> Saccharin created the foundation for many low-calorie and sugar-free products around the world. It is still used in tabletop sweeteners, baked goods, jams, chewing gum, canned fruit, candy, dessert toppings and salad dressings.

Saccharin contains only one-eighth of a calorie per teaspoon, and is approximately 300 times sweeter than sugar. Today, saccharin is available in both powdered and liquid forms, <u>sold without the cancer warning</u>, and is being reintroduced into food products as **safe**. If you must use an artificial sweetener, I personally recommend saccharin use over aspartame and sucralose, due to the respective methanol and chlorine.

Stevia—Is It Safe?

I receive many inquiries about the safety of stevia. So, *"Is it safe?"* Absolutely. Not only is it safe, it may even be good for you.

Stevia is 250 to 300 times sweeter than sugar. It is isolated and purified from the leaves of the stevia plant. Stevia has been used as a traditional remedy for diabetes and gum disease among the indigenous people of Paraguay and other South American countries for over 1,500 recorded years. (Who knows how many years prior to the records?) Preliminary scientific evidence (performed by independent researchers) shows stevia may indeed improve the function of cells required for insulin production in the pancreas, and may also improve glucose tolerance in people with diabetes. According to the generations of people who have used stevia as a part of their daily diet, stevia has also been proven to regulate blood sugar.

Unlike other sweeteners, stevia has been reported to possess anti-viral activity. Preliminary evidence suggests that stevia possesses blood pressure-lowering properties and may be a useful treatment for hypertension.

THE NEED TO TEST: Prior to the onslaught of chemical sugar substitutes, before now the need to "test" stevia for negative health effects has never been necessary after 1,500 years of use, just as we find little need to test the herbs basil or thyme. People who have used stevia for generations in South America, Japan, China and Indonesian countries do not use stevia as often or in the same quantities as modern consumers use artificial sweeteners. Further research will be required for stevia safety, though, because as stevia becomes more competitive on the modern sweetener market, it will become more of a threat to the chemical sweetener companies. After years of political scrutiny and stonewalling in Europe, October 2004, stevia was finally approved by the European Commission for use as a sweetener.

I feel stevia is a much safer sweetener alternative compared to the artificial chemicals created in corporate laboratories, especially for use during pregnancy, for children and for diabetics who stand to benefit from its effects on glucose. Of course, the key to eating anything properly, whether chemical food replacements or one-hundred percent natural foods, is to be moderate in its use.

Tips To Avoid Bitterness:
*Try different brands of stevia before giving up on it, as some are milder-tasting than others
*Stevia is much sweeter than Equal®, Splenda®, and the other chemical sweeteners, so use significantly less than you might think is necessary
*Start with using one-quarter the amount of stevia as you'd use of the other chemicals and increase as needed. It comes in both liquid and powdered form.

Your Healthy Choices

The following is an alphabetized list of the best natural choices for sweeteners that are safer for long-term health as opposed to the refined sugars and the artificial chemical sweeteners. Remember nothing is without consequence. <u>Natural is always a better choice, but all of these alternatives should be eaten in moderation, as most can impact blood sugar levels</u>. It is best to use *any type* of sweetener, even the all-natural ones, sparingly, *if at all*, with the optimal choice being to savor the natural flavors in your food and resist the urge to add extra sweetness.

<u>Natural sweetener choices</u> (besides saccharin and stevia):
1. Barley Malt
2. Brown Rice Syrup
3. Date Sugar
4. Honey (raw unpasteurized honey is best)
5. Maple Syrup and Maple Sugar
6. Molasses
7. Sorghum
8. Sucanat

"<u>Grey area</u>" sweeteners (those that are natural, yet are either slightly altered in laboratory processing or naturally tend to spike

blood sugar):
1. Fructose
2. Fruit Juice Concentrate
3. Sugar Alcohols
4. Tagatose
5. Turbinado® Sugar

New natural sweeteners:
1. Lo Han
2. Tastes Like Sugar®
3. Trehalose
4. Yacón®

A Quick Explanation Of Natural Sweetener Choices:

BARLEY MALT: Barley malt is a thick, dark, slow-digesting sweetener made from sprouted, roasted barley grain with a nutty, malt-like flavor. Barley malt can be bought in granular form or as syrup. It is called "malt" because maltose is the sugar that occurs when starch in the barley sprouts. Barley malt is used in brewing beer, and some say barley malt is to beer as grapes are to wine. It is ideally suited to brewing for many reasons:

1. Malted barley has a high balance of enzymes for converting its starch into simple sugars
2. It also contains protein, which is needed for yeast nutrition

Barley malt extract is used medicinally as a bulking agent to promote bowel regularity. Because the malt comes from sprouted barley, the malt can be concentrated into a soluble fiber, so it has laxative qualities similar to psyllium, oats and the pectin in fruits. Beneficial bacteria in the colon use barley fiber for food. Barley malt is helpful in chronic constipation, irritable bowel syndrome, diverticulosis, hiatal hernia and diabetes. Soluble fiber can even lower cholesterol ten percent to fifteen percent.

Because barley malt is an actual food sugar, it should be refrigerated for extended storage.

BROWN RICE SYRUP: Rice syrup is made by slow-cooking brown rice until it develops thick sweet syrup. Few people have allergies to rice, so this offers an alternative sweetener choice for consumers with allergies or asthma, particularly children. Rice syrup has a light flavor because it is a food. There is no need to refrigerate rice syrup. If the syrup hardens, simply run the jar under warm water.

DATE SUGAR: Date sugar is made by dehydrating and pulverizing dates. The date fruit has a high concentration of naturally-occurring sugars. This particular sugar does not dissolve well, but it is acceptable for cooking and baking. Date sugar should be stored in a cool, dry place.

Date sugar is high in fiber and contains a long list of vitamins and minerals, including iron. Substitute one cup date sugar for each cup granulated sugar for a better choice of sweeteners.

HONEY: For centuries, honey has been referred to as "nature's gold." After gathering the nectar from flowers and flowering plants, bees return to the hive and process the nectar as honey. (Local bee pollen, the precursor to honey in the hive, is great for allergies.) The flavor of the honey reflects the flower. Sources commonly include buckwheat, blackberry, heather, clover, orange blossoms, wildflowers and sage. To process raw honey, remove it from its wax comb, strain or heat and filter. The downside to this process is that heating the honey destroys many of its natural enzymes and nutrients. For this reason, I highly recommend you seek out a source of raw honey, which is a much healthier alternative to the commercial pasteurized honey in most supermarkets. You can find raw honey in some health food stores or from local farmers. Caution: most labels warn not to feed infants and toddlers honey because they cannot process it properly yet.

Honey should be stored in a dry place. If the honey begins to crystallize, place the jar in a pot of hot water until the sugar crystals dissolve. Be careful not to make the water too hot or you risk damaging the nutrients. Honey contains the following nutrients: protein, thiamin, riboflavin, niacin, vitamin C, calcium and iron. Topical application of honey to infected wounds is an ancient remedy, and one that has been confirmed by many scientific studies.

MAPLE SYRUP AND MAPLE SUGAR: Thirty-five to fifty gallons of maple tree sap boil down to one gallon of maple syrup. Classified by color and flavor, the lighter the syrup color (Grade A), the lighter the flavor. The grades of syrup have more to do with taste than quality. The darker the color, the longer the syrup has usually boiled, shifting it further from its original state. Maple syrups and sugars should be refrigerated.

MOLASSES: The liquid that is spun out of refining cane sugar is molasses. Molasses is twenty percent to twenty-five percent water, fifty percent sugar and ten percent ash, with some protein and organic acids remaining. Molasses is graded by color and sugar content, with the lighter color containing more sugar. So look for the darker grades. Because of its very strong flavor, molasses is used mainly in baking and should be kept cool or refrigerated.

SORGHUM: Sorghum is a grain related to millet. It is processed into a sweetener by crushing the plant stalks and boiling the extracted juice into syrup. Sorghum is comparable to molasses but is much lighter and milder tasting. Sorghum should be refrigerated.

SUCANAT®—**Su**gar **Ca**ne **Nat**ural: Sucanat is a natural granulated sweetener with a higher nutrition level and a lower sugar level than refined sugar (88.3% vs.99.9%). Fresh cane juice is pressed from the sugar cane stalk and then dehydrated through a co-crystallization process. It is through this process that Sucanat granules are formed. Sucanat granules are an improvement over bleached sugar crystals in shape and function. Unlike processed sugar crystals, Sucanat granules are round, porous and easily compressed, and can be used in the "sugar bowl" as refined sugars are used, but are a much healthier alternative. My sons were raised on Sucanat in our sugar bowl.

Product qualities include:

- No additives or preservatives
- Lower sugar level than refined sugar
- One-for-one replacement for refined white sugar, brown sugar and honey
- Homogeneous blending
- Natural rich flavor
- Compressible
- Excellent consistency and texture in baked goods
- Instant solubility

Note: Liquid natural sweeteners (barley malt, brown rice syrup, honey and maple syrup) can be stored at room temperature in the original packaging, but should be refrigerated after opening. Dry, powdered alternative sweeteners should be stored in a dry place at room temperature. Fruit juice concentrates should remain frozen until ready to use.

A Quick Explanation Of The "Grey Area" Sweeteners:

<u>FRUCTOSE</u>: Fructose becomes a simple sugar by refining corn syrup or extracting beet sugar. Because it breaks down more slowly in the body than sucrose, it has a somewhat lesser effect on blood-sugar levels, but it does not provide any nutritional

benefits. Also known as levulose and fruit sugar, fructose is the sweetest of all the simple sugars. Fruits naturally contain between one percent and seven percent fructose, although some fruits have much higher amounts. Fructose makes up about forty percent of the dry weight of honey. It is also available in crystalline form, but its sweetness rapidly declines when dissolved in water. Some people react badly to fructose, so it is not a recommended option for those who need to restrict sugar intake.

In fact, I do not recommend fructose as an acceptable form of sugar for anyone despite its acceptance in many nutritional circles. The reasons for this are many:

- Nearly all simple sugars, including fructose, are metabolized rapidly, which disrupts insulin and blood sugar levels
- Fructose contributes to most chronic illness
- One of the primary ways that people ingest fructose is in the form of high-fructose corn syrup (HFCS), which is used to sweeten everything from soda to canned fruits to chewing gum. HFCS contains similar amounts of both fructose and glucose (see below), whereas sucrose (table sugar) is a larger sugar molecule that is metabolized in the intestine into glucose and fructose

The digestive and absorptive processes for glucose and fructose are different. Unlike glucose, which the body uses for energy, when you consume large amounts of fructose, it supplies a relatively unregulated source of fuel for the liver to convert to fat and cholesterol. Fructose converts to fat more than any other sugar.

Further, most fructose is consumed in a liquid form, which significantly magnifies its negative metabolic effects. The devastation it has on our biology would be significantly lessened if it was slowly absorbed from solid food, but most fructose is consumed in soft drinks and fruit juices. This is one type of sweetener I don't advise anyone to add to his or her diet. Note: This does NOT apply as strictly to the fructose ingested in whole fruits. Eating balanced amounts of natural fruits provides less "adulterated" fructose than manufactured forms of fructose products, posing less of a problem for most people. Caution is advised for people with diabetes or obesity.

FRUIT JUICE CONCENTRATE: This sweetener undergoes little processing, but most people don't think about sweetening with fruit concentrates. It can be used to sweeten more products than you'd think, such as cookies, candy, cereal and sodas. Fruit juice concentrate is usually made from a concentrate of pineapple, pear, peach or clarified grape juice. They can be used much more safely than artificial sweeteners when sweetening gelatin, unsweetened powdered drinks and fruit smoothies.

Most fruit juice concentrates are frozen, so keep in the freezer until ready for use.

SUGAR ALCOHOLS: I am not a fan of sugar alcohols extracted from their natural sources. Sugar alcohols are actually made from sugar. Part of their structure chemically resembles sugar and part is similar to alcohol. To complicate matters more, these sweeteners are neither sugars nor alcohols—they are best described as a sugar byproduct <u>refined by nature, processed by man</u>. Sugar alcohols fall into a "grey area" in the sweetener arena because they are actually carbohydrates (starches) more than they are sugars. They are typically used cup-for-cup in the same amount as refined sugar, but they each vary in sweetness, ranging from half as sweet to as sweet as sugar. Sugar alcohols blend well with other sugars, so they are commonly added to products such as gums, candies and mints, toothpaste and mouthwash. <u>Please keep in mind, these "grey area" sugar alcohols can give people gastric distress if consumed in excess.</u>

Included in this group are:

- Erythritol
- Hydrogenated Starch Hydrolysates
- Isomalt
- Lactitol
- Maltitol
- Mannitol
- Sorbitol
- Xylitol

Sugar alcohols are used in a wide range of low-calorie, low-fat and sugar-free foods from baked goods to frozen dairy desserts since they provide bulk without all the calories of sugar. Sugar alcohols do not commonly promote tooth decay, so are used in toothpastes, mouthwashes, breath mints and pharmaceuticals such as cough syrups, cough drops and throat lozenges.

THE DOWNSIDE OF SUGAR ALCOHOLS: Some of the sugar alcohols that are not absorbed in the blood are broken down into fatty acids in the large intestine. People on low-carbohydrate diets or who have diabetes may not respond well to the sugar alcohols in place of sugar because some people report that sugar alcohols act as "trigger foods," causing carb cravings or binges.

Since the intestine does absorb the sugar alcohols, excessive use can cause gas or laxative effects similar to reactions to beans and certain high-fiber foods. Such symptoms depend, of course, on an individual's sensitivity, health status, and what other foods are eaten at the same time. Another positive way to look at it—your body may be showing you its limit on how much sugar it really needs by "kicking out" too much.

The table below provides a summary of each of the different sugar alcohols currently used in U.S. food products. Nutrition labels include them as either "Sugar Alcohols" or under their individual name.

<u>1. Erythritol</u> is an odorless white, crystalline powder with a clean sweet taste approximately seventy percent as sweet as sugar. Like most sugar alcohols, erythritol does not promote tooth decay. It has approximately seven percent to thirteen percent the calories of other sugar alcohols and five percent the calories of sugar. Because erythritol is rapidly absorbed in the small intestine and rapidly eliminated by the body (within twenty-four hours), laxative side effects are sometimes associated with excessive use.

<u>2. Hydrogenated Starch Hydrolysates</u> (HSH) are a mixture of sorbitol, maltitol and hydrogenated oligosaccharides. Depending on the type of HSH desired (the maltitol and sorbitol content can be varied), the sweetness of HSH varies from twenty-five percent to fifty percent that of sucrose. HSH sweeteners are used in a wide variety of candies, gums and mints. Also known as maltitol syrup and hydrogenated glucose syrup. Just remember to read your labels!

<u>3. Isomalt</u> is a complex carb (one of the better sugars) and approximately forty-five percent to sixty-five percent as sweet as sucrose. Isomalt is used in candies, gums, ice cream, jams and jellies, fillings and frostings, beverages and baked products. As a sweetener/bulking agent, it has no off-flavors and works well in combination with other sweeteners.

<u>4. Lactitol</u> is a sweet-tasting complex carb (another good sugar) derived from lactose. Lactitol provides the bulk and texture of sugar with half the calories. Thirty percent to forty percent as sweet as sucrose, it is used in: baked goods, chewing gum, confections and frostings, frozen dairy desserts and mixes, candy, jams and jellies.

5. Maltitol is a complex carb produced by the hydrogenation of maltose, the sugar found naturally in sprouted grain. It occurs widely in nature, for example, in chicory and roasted malt. About 0.9 times as sweet as sucrose with similar sweetness and body, maltitol is suitable for many kinds of candies, gums and mints, and is particularly good for candy coating.

6. Mannitol is a simple carb (simple sugar), approximately 0.7 times as sweet as sucrose. Used as a bulking agent in powdered foods and as a *dusting agent for chewing gum* (interesting!), excessive consumption of more than twenty grams a day may have a laxative effect. Mannitol has been removed from the GRAS (Generally Recognized As Safe) list, and is regulated as an interim "food additive." This means that its current use is considered safe, but some questions have been raised that must be resolved to fully determine what limitations, if any, should be imposed. Mannitol is permitted for use in many countries, including the United States.

Sorbitol (see below) and mannitol are readily converted in the body to fructose and glucose. The problem with these sweeteners is they are slowly absorbed from the intestines and may produce a laxative or gaseous effect, and may affect blood sugar levels more than the other sugar alcohols, so they may not be the best choice for diabetics.

7. Sorbitol is another simple carb sixty percent as sweet as sucrose. Excessive consumption of more than fifty to eighty grams a day may have a laxative effect. Sorbitol is also a sugar alcohol the body uses slowly. It is called a nutritive sweetener because it actually has four calories in every gram, just like table sugar. Sorbitol is found naturally in fruits and is an ingredient in many sugar-free gums, sugar-free breath mints and dietetic candies.

> Did you know that sorbitol is also produced by the body?
> Too much sorbitol in your cells can cause damage, though.
> Diabetic retinopathy and neuropathy may be related to too
> much sorbitol in the cells of the eyes and nerves.

CAUTION: Some foods contain sugars that are absorbed slowly, such as fructose in fruit juice or sorbitol in low-calorie sweets. Through a process called osmosis, these unabsorbed sugars hold onto water in the intestines, which sometimes leads to diarrhea. By reading labels, people with chronic non-infectious diarrhea can easily avoid fruit juice, fructose and sorbitol to see if this eliminates the problem.

8. Xylitol seems to be the "favored child" of the sugar alcohols. It is a simple carb, though, extracted from birch tree pulp. The wood sugar "xylose" was first hydrogenated to produce xylitol in 1891 by the German chemist Emil Fischer. Xylitol has been used since the 1960s in the Soviet Union, Germany, Switzerland and Japan as a favored sweetener for diabetics. Xylitol is also used intravenously for patients with impaired glucose tolerance, i.e. for trauma, burns, and in diabetic and insulin-resistant states.

Xylitol is a naturally-occurring sweetener also found in:

- Raspberries
- Strawberries
- Plums
- Corn
- Endive
- Mushrooms

Xylitol does not require insulin to metabolize in the body and does not promote tooth decay. Xylitol has the same sweetness, bulk and caloric value as sucrose, so it is one of the most popular sweetener alternatives used in candies, chewing gum and natural-ingredient toothpastes, foods such as gum drops and hard candy, and in pharmaceuticals and oral health products.

Because xylitol helps prevent plaque and cavities, it is a better choice for sugarless gums than aspartame or sucralose. But in the long term, you are better off using neither sugar nor natural unprocessed sugars. As with most sugar alcohols, consumers with hypoglycemia, Candida or diabetes may react negatively to xylitol.

SOMETHING TO WATCH FOR: Kelly Goyen, Founder/CEO of Empirical Labs has observed children with AD/HD react in the same fashion to Xylitol as to aspartame or high doses of refined sugar. "Xylitol passes through the blood-brain barrier," Goyen states, "and we have observed at our laboratory that after using Xylitol, hypersensitive children become more 'active' shortly after use."

TAGATOSE: Labeled Naturlose® for use in pharmaceuticals and toothpaste, tagatose hopes to "take over the market," according to marketing experts. Tagatose, discovered in 1981, is a partially-digestible sugar made from whey. It claims to be all natural, low calorie, and almost as sweet as sucrose. It is being studied for unsafe effects on infants and pregnancy, however. Currently, the license contract for tagatose is tied up in arbitration and its patent as a food additive expires in 2008.

Even though fertility issues are under scrutiny, company executives for Sperix (Naturlose manufacturer) claim their sweetener product enhances fertility and high pregnancy rates in laboratory rats fed tagatose, prevents biofilm (bacteria that forms on teeth and medical instruments) and enhances key blood factors critical to fighting anemia.

Tagatose is synergistic with other sweeteners and can improve texture and "mouth-feel" in sugar-free products. Potential uses for tagatose include candies, gums and mints, ready-to-eat cereal, ice cream and baked goods. The Kellogg Company, Battle Creek, Michigan, has received a patent for the use of tagatose in ready-to-eat cereal and other foods.

TURBINADO® SUGAR: This is the light brown crystalline substance removed from molasses during the first separation during processing, moving from a complex sugar (that doesn't pass into the blood stream) to a simple sugar (that passes into the blood). Although Turbinado contains trace nutrients, it is identical to white sugar in the way it is absorbed by the body. Turbinado should be stored in a cool, dry place.

A Quick Explanation Of New Sweeteners:

LO HAN: The Chinese plant Lo Han Guo Siraitia grosvenorii is a perennial vine in the cucumber, melon, squash and gourd family. Lo Han fruits are used both inside and outside the People's Republic of China as a food, beverage and traditional medicine. Although millions of Lo Han fruits are consumed worldwide each year, Lo Han fruits in Europe and the United States are mostly sold by Chinese grocery and herb stores. The current uses and potential of Lo Han Guo are as a food, seasoning, beverage or non-caloric sweetener plant.

The Chinese book <u>Fruit as Medicine</u> (Dai and Liu, 1986) reports these fruits are used for heat stroke (with thirst), acute and chronic throat inflammation, chronic cough, constipation in the aged, and as a sugar substitute for diabetics. In general, you boil or simmer the fruit in water and drink it as an herb tea. As a sugar substitute in cooking, the fruits may be simmered into a thick juice and added to food. The prepared block form called "Luohanguo Chongji" is reported to be a popular treatment for colds in China.

<u>TASTES LIKE SUGAR</u>®: Here's some new sweetener research: *mung beans that sweeten.*

Kelly Goyen, CEO/Founder of Empirical Labs, has created an all-natural sweetener called Tastes Like Sugar made from inulin, mung bean extract, and fermented green papaya, a natural digestive enzyme to complete digestion of sugars and carbohydrates. "Everyone who has tested Tastes Like Sugar has raved about it," states Goyen. Tastes Like Sugar does not alter blood sugar in diabetics, and tests have shown no change in mental or physical behavior in hyperactive children. The sweetener is all-natural with no compromising additives, and is fifty times sweeter than sucrose.

Inulin, the first ingredient in Tastes Like Sugar, is a chemical believed to improve blood lipid levels and is currently being studied as a pre-cancer preventative nutrient. Recent animal research shows that inulin prevents adverse precancerous changes in the colon. Inulin is recommended for diabetics, and because it is not absorbed into the bloodstream, it does not affect blood sugar levels. Inulin has a mildly sweet taste, and is filling like starchy foods. It is a preferred food for the lactobacilli in the intestine and can improve the balance of friendly bacteria in the bowel.

Mung beans are the most consumed sprout on Earth, grown and used extensively in Asia. Mungs are actually twenty percent protein and contain vitamins A, B, C and E, calcium, iron, magnesium, potassium, and complex amino acids. Perhaps the most exciting of the sprouts, mungs are sweet when ripened and appear to be a healthy alternative to chemical sweetener blends.

For more information on Tastes Like Sugar, email <u>orders@empirical-labs.com</u> or call (970) 461-3780. Suzanne Somer's SomerSweet® also uses the mung bean as a natural sweetening ingredient, and I also recommend SomerSweet® as a safe alternative sweetener.

TREHALOSE®: Trehalose is one of the most interesting new sweeteners on the market today, and I felt it was worth including in this chapter primarily due to the "honesty in advertising" the company has expressed about their new product. I should probably classify Trehalose as a grey-area sweetener because no one really knows enough about it to date, yet it appears a solid product backed by sound science. This sweetener is a disaccharide (a good carb) with two glucose molecules (a better choice for diabetics because it is a complex carb), but what impressed me the most is the company's honesty in admitting that <u>Trehalose is fully digested and metabolized</u>. Finally, someone admits their sweetener is digested! This is the most "natural" form of sugar metabolism.

Cargill Health & Food Technologies, makers of Trehalose, markets the new sweetener for sports drinks. In November 2003, PacificHealth Laboratories, Woodbridge, NJ, announced the launch of a ready-to-drink form of its sports drink, Accelerade®. It provides the energy (from complex sugar carbs) needed in sports, according to the company representatives. I'd rather see an athlete drink pure water for body restoration, but Trehalose appears a better choice than the other artificial sweeteners, and that's all athletes have to choose from when it comes to low-carb sports drinks and energy bars.

Trehalose is found naturally in honey, mushrooms and other foods. One aspect I am concerned about, though, is Trehalose is commercially produced from cornstarch, which can cause allergic reactions and stomach irritations in some people. Its functions include coloring adjunct, flavor enhancer, humectant, nutritive sweetener, stabilizer, thickener and texturizer. Trehalose can also protect and preserve food's cell structure, which can help maintain food texture during freezing and thawing. Trehalose is found in candies, gums and mints, processed foods, such as dried vegetables and fruits, and dairy and fruit products.

YACÓN®: Yacón is not a commercial sweetener yet, but look for this natural sweetener coming to the American market in the near future. A distant relative of the sunflower, Yacón grows from Venezuela to Argentina in small farm orchards in the inner mountain valleys. Yacón is a natural plant root with a rich sweet flavor. In spite of its sweetness, Yacón is composed of complex plant sugars, so it will not penetrate the intestines and contribute to weight gain. This is also a plus for diabetics because Yacón contains traces of inulin.

Yacón can be eaten raw, just like a fruit, and once the roots have been dried in the sun, they become sweeter. Hopefully it will be available in America soon.

Sweetening Tips

Don't use any added sugars at all. Ideally, learn to appreciate the natural sweetness of your food. The more natural the food, the sweeter the taste. This is always the best option!

Use more spices and herbs when preparing meals instead of adding sweetness.

If eating a dessert, choose a natural fruit. Apples, cheese, grapes, fruits and nuts are common desserts in European countries. If you must sweeten, select from the safe sweetener list.

Honey can be used to replace sugar in a recipe: 3/4 cup of honey can replace one cup of sugar in a recipe. However, you will have to reduce the liquid by one-half cup for each cup of honey you add to the recipe.

If you want to cut down on your total intake of sugar, consider decreasing all sugars—white, brown, powdered, raw, as well as honey. You could limit your intake of foods high in sugar to once a week rather than eating sweets daily. Another significant reduction in sugar could be made by adding only one-half to one-third the amount of sugar or honey called for in a recipe. You will be surprised how good cookies taste with half the sugar. There are also many healthy recipes out there that call for no added sugar at all!

Instead of trying so hard to sweeten your food, wouldn't it be refreshing if you were satisfied with fresh berries or a simple piece of fruit? Maybe this should be your goal—to return your taste buds to normal stimulation. So, have an apple or a cup of berries before you read the next chapter!

CHAPTER 5

How To Eliminate Toxic Chemicals From Your Body

After more than two decades of consuming diet sweeteners, the average human being is getting fatter, disease is at epidemic levels, and emotional stress is ruining people's lives at younger and younger ages. With excess weight an important factor in the onset of cancer, heart disease, and diabetes, it now appears we are facing a health crisis spreading across the face of this planet. In every country where diet sweeteners are sold, research indicates an increase in illness inevitably follows. As other artificial sweeteners compete for the number one spot in the "diet" market and sweetener blends intensify these toxins, consumers must change their dietary habits to secure a healthier lifestyle.

I wrote in my first book, <u>Sweet Poison: *How The World's Most Popular Artificial Sweetener Is Killing Us*</u>, how I cured a "fatal" case of Grave's Disease by removing aspartame completely from my diet. In my second book, <u>Ten Steps To Detoxification: *A Nutrition and Diet Regimen Designed To Cleanse Your Body of Toxic Chemicals,*</u> I explain the step-by-step process I created to restore my health from Grave's Disease based on my professional background as a Hazardous Waste and Emergency Response engineer and nutritionist. In essence, I clean up the body's inner environment as an engineer cleans the outer environment. In this chapter, I share what I learned with you.

After helping hundreds of people around the world deal with chemical poisoning, I developed my Detoxification Program to remove toxins from body tissues and restore the nutrients that toxic by-products destroy inside the body. Modern medicine has led human beings to the "take-a-pill-or-cut-it-out" mentality for almost every modern health symptom, but more and more people are personally discovering that this approach alone cannot cure disease. If anything, we just keep getting sicker and more physically tired until our bodies eventually give in to disease. Curing illness and degenerative diseases as in times past might be considered old-fashioned and ineffective when compared to today's high-tech standards, but our physical bodies haven't changed over time nor have the effects of disease, just the magnitude of modern treatments and the chemicals that cause illness. It's essential that human beings remember that the roots of disease and their cures are as old-fashioned as the body itself. This is the basis for my Detoxification Program.

Become aware of those around you who have chemical diets or have been exposed to radiation or heavy metals, and notice their health symptoms. Headaches may have them down - again. Maybe it's a migraine this time, yet they'll tell you they <u>never</u> had a migraine before now. Seizures may be a recurring problem, and they're frustrated because they'll tell you they <u>never</u> had seizures before either, and their doctor can find no cause for sudden life-threatening conditions. Do you know anyone who has recently been diagnosed with Lupus, Grave's Disease, Fibromyalgia, Chronic Fatigue Syndrome, or Diabetes? Or maybe your children are showing signs of hyperactivity, yet <u>never</u> had a behavior problem before now?

114

The U.N. World Health Organization is warning nations that a worldwide epidemic of diabetes will soon be a reality, yet no one has the answer to "why?" Degenerative diseases are at epidemic levels today, and doctors have no clue as to the causes. Trillions of dollars are being spent on pharmaceuticals to control the symptoms of disease and the threat of war chemicals, but no long-term cures have been discovered by traditional medicine nor have been proven to be safe for long-term health and wellness. Chemical sugar substitutes are now taking over our food supply, and are found in simple drinking water, children's medications, painkillers – as well as thousands of products from gums to cereals. Modern doctors have no answers for the increase in degenerative diseases, and debilitating illnesses are occurring at younger and younger ages. These "Western" disease syndromes are now appearing for the first time in other countries exposed to our modern diets and threats of chemical warfare.

The dangers of poisoning from the chemicals in our food supply and medications have been a well-guarded secret in America. Traditional doctors and many alternative doctors are not properly informed about the adverse effects this myriad of chemicals has on human health. But the research and history of chemical poisoning is conclusive as a cause of illness and toxic reactions in the human body. The harmful effects to children are some of the greatest tragedies of modern times.

After more than fifty years of manmade chemicals saturating our food supply and now with the threat of radiation and chemical poisoning from war and terrorism, the number of victims is rapidly piling up. People are figuring out for themselves that chemical exposure is at the root of many of their health problems. Patients are teaching their doctors about this nutritional peril, and many are healing themselves with little to no support from traditional medicine. This trend has become more evident over the last few years. Even large corporations are picking up on this.

These corporations are becoming financially strapped by worker health insurance claims. They are now investigating prevention programs to keep their employees on the job. Personal wellness to <u>prevent</u> disease (rather than waiting until sickness strikes) is actually becoming a successful business strategy!

Pharmaceutical medicines do not cure the underlying <u>causes</u> of disease. They merely suppress the symptoms and end up expensive in the long term. Prescribed drugs are actually creating more adverse symptoms themselves. Then tragically, more drugs are prescribed to counteract those side effects. So many new medications are coming onto the American market each week, most human beings can't keep track of their long-term effects or the many interactions the drugs may have with one another.

> The modern American approach to medicine - administering drugs instead of healthy prevention - is like treating a headache as an "aspirin deficiency disease." The causes of disease must be determined before the cures can be found. The most effective way to reverse disease symptoms is often by removing the underlying cause – modern manmade chemicals saturating our food supply, our water stores, our pharmaceuticals, and our living environments.

My Detoxification Program can help improve your health and possibly change your life forever. It changed mine! You can regain control of your life in "Ten Basic Steps."

I am not minimizing the seriousness of genetic or degenerative diseases, but in many cases, until the cause of a disease is determined, the cure cannot be permanently put into place.

More than likely if you are suffering from health symptoms your doctor cannot identify, then you are reacting to an environmental cause - something outside of your body that's penetrating inside. This is good news actually, because if your doctor cannot "see" any physical damage yet, then it's not too late to turn your nagging disease symptoms around and restore good health. This means you do not have to live the rest of your life dependent on expensive prescribed medications, medicines that can be toxic in the long run, creating even more health problems and dependencies. (And if we have another global war, can you be assured you can get your prescriptions refilled anyway?)

If you begin preventative detoxification procedures before chemical exposure, then your body will be prepared to defend its immune system more efficiently if chemical exposure were to occur. Begin a chemical-free lifestyle today.

The Ten Steps

1. Identify and remove the cause of your health symptoms
2. Learn to "read" your body. Begin recording any health changes
3. Get a hair analysis
4. Be happy with yourself
5. Detoxify your body
6. Restore depleted nutrients
7. Exercise and get plenty of rest
8. Eat 75% raw foods at every meal
9. Drink water, water, water
10. Get control of your life

Step One: Identify And Remove The Cause Of Your Health Symptoms

Specifically, remove all chemicals from your diet and environment immediately. Become aware of the chemical additives in all your foods. Really KNOW what is going into your body at all times. Don't cheat yourself.

I tell people to look for their body's weakest link, which is usually a genetic weakness, such as the colon, the heart, etc. This is where toxins within your body will be "noticed" first because this is the most vulnerable part of your physical make-up. Toxins like mercury or radiation will absorb into your weakest link first, breaking it down faster. By removing all chemicals from your diet and environment, you can focus on strengthening your weaknesses rather than tearing them down.

Purify your environment as much as possible. Remove any toxins from both inside and outside your body. Inspect your house and place of employment for:

1. Old pipes
2. Leaking insulation
3. Unsafe drinking water
4. Dusty air vents
5. Pesticides
6. Radon
7. Mold
8. Chemicals upstream or upwind
9. Air quality
10. Toxic metals
11. Leaky power sources

Read food labels. Most people first look at the price of a food product and then glance to see if it's reduced-calorie or fat-free. Instead, look for the natural content with the fewest ingredients. Minimize buying processed and packaged foods. The closer to its natural state (as in raw vegetables), the more it will feed your cells. Metals, such as inorganic aluminum and nickel along with a variety of toxic chemicals like methanol found in aspartame and chlorine in sucralose, are used in the manufacturing of foods. No one needs to <u>eat</u> these chemicals. The manufacturing and packaging of foods removes natural vitamins and minerals, too. Many times, artificial fillers are injected into foods to stretch profits. "Enrichment" isn't the same to the body as "natural." <u>The purer the food, the fewer the ingredients.</u>

Additives you want to avoid:

1. Aspartame
2. Autolyzed yeast
3. All food colorings
4. All hydrogenated and partially hydrogenated oils
5. Calcium caseinate
6. Gelatin
7. Glutamate
8. Glutamic acid
9. Hydrolyzed protein
10. Monopotassium glutamate
11. Monosodium glutamate
12. Sodium caseinate
13. Textured protein
14. Yeast extract

Don't overindulge on fast foods so you won't have to give them up altogether. Just be aware of how much and how often you "indulge" on them, and try to minimize the chemicals you are eating. Be picky about the fast food stops you make, and choose the better quality in all food choices. If you want to order a pizza, for example, order one from an authentic Italian restaurant that makes their pizzas fresh with natural ingredients rather than ordering one from popular food chains replete with chemical-processed-assembly-line foods saturated with chemical preservatives and lifeless oils.

Step Two: Learn To Read Your Body And Begin Recording Any Health Changes

Do you remember the last time you really felt good? Think about when you first started feeling ill and when your first health symptoms occurred. Go backwards in time day-by-day, month-by-month, or year-by-year until you can stop at the point when you started feeling sick. This is where you start over. You may have been through a tough emotional time, or you might have been very ill with a high fever. But were you drinking diet colas or living downstream from a factory? So, pick up where you got off-track and start over at that point.

Once you have removed all chemicals from your diet and environment, and have read all your labels for hidden food chemicals, notice if your health symptoms disappear. A woman in London who drank diet colas for many years emailed me with her story. For the past nine years, she had been sick. She began having seizures; sporadically at first and small in impact. Then they began to occur more often, with more intensity. Over a six-month period, she was having two seizures a day. She lost her memory during the seizures, and they affected her work. In and out of doctor's offices, no one could find anything wrong with her. Sound familiar?

Desperate to find answers her doctors could not give her, she read my first book <u>Sweet Poison</u> and got off all aspartame. Within three days, her recurring seizures stopped. If she accidentally got into hidden aspartame in any form, she would have another seizure. The medication her doctors prescribed for her began to cause seizures, too. Now aspartame-free, having detoxed, and continuously supplementing with the specific vitamins and nutrients specified for her individual needs, she no longer needs her medication. Her doctors thought she was crazy to get off the prescribed medicine, as that was the only solution they had for her unexplained seizures. (I'm not recommending anyone stop their prescribed medications without consulting their physician, but I do advise alternative ways to lessen dependency on medications that mask health symptoms rather then treating the cause of disease.)

Aspartame-free and seizure-free, this young woman restored her health day by day. She noticed that not only were her seizures gone, but she was able to sleep throughout the night for the first time in years, her hair, skin, and nails returned to normal, her mood swings were gone, her weight dropped and her energy level increased. Her memory is now sharper, and her sex drive returned.

Take the time to read your body. Learn your limits. Notice if you have more energy when detoxing various body chemicals, or if you sleep better and have better dreams. Note if you look and feel younger. Do you have more vigor and are you in better control of your life? Give yourself credit - **you** can control your life again, the natural way.

Step Three: Get A Hair Analysis

As I discovered through my personal recovery from disease, I couldn't fight what I couldn't see. It wasn't probable that I would cure my disease if no one knew the cause. The hair analysis is the best "road map" to see a history of what's going on inside of your body. Drug and chemical residues within the body remain embedded in the protein of the hair as it grows. Drugs such as cocaine and heroin may not be detected in urine several days after use, yet these drugs will show up in a hair analysis months later. Hair has the advantage of long-term memory. It's a permanent record, like tree rings. A three-inch strand of hair will give a six-month history of what's going on in the body since head hair grows at a rate of about a half an inch a month.

I recommend *everyone* have at least one hair analysis in his or her lifetime to "see" what your body is in need of. A hair analysis is the highest caliber of laboratory science a Certified Nutritionist or Doctor of Natural Medicine can use. You can go to my website www.hairanalysisprogram.com or www. detoxprogram.net to learn more.

The hair holds an imprint of all vitamin and mineral levels in the body and reflects minute levels of toxins deposited in the tissues. As human beings become more polluted, a hair analysis can also detect specific toxins that have stored in the body. It's a great diagnostic tool. Before taking any vitamin and mineral supplements, consult a Certified Nutritionist for your specific health needs. Every individual is different, and a hair analysis can identify personal nutritional needs.

With a background in environmental engineering, I would not be able to make an accurate decision on how to clean up a toxic spill without performing a soil or water analysis of the polluted area. So it is with a hair analysis - the hair provides the best view of what is within the body.

Many traditional medical doctors criticize the hair analysis as not being a respected diagnostic test for human beings, not measuring up to blood tests, urine tests, MRIs or CAT scans. But I believe their protests are sourced to a lack of nutritional education and background needed to interpret the hair tests properly. In police work, forensic scientists use hair tests that stand up in court, attesting to their validity.

The key to any good lab analysis is in its interpretation, and without a thorough background in nutrition and in the sources of disease, typical lab tests are less effective in long term healing. You might witness this when you go to the doctor with mysterious health symptoms, yet receive no answers as to why you feel sick and the lab results show nothing there. Doctors prescribe "medications" to help relieve your symptoms, but don't fix the underlying problem.

Step Four: Be Happy With Yourself

Ask yourself WHY you are using:

1. Sugar-free diet products?
2. Alcohol?
3. Prescribed and over-the-counter medications?
4. Have you had your old mercury fillings removed?
5. How long have you been refilling that prescription without question?
6. When did you begin changing your diet from natural foods to an artificial chemical diet?
7. Are you diabetic?
8. Do you give sugar-free foods to your children because you think keeping them off sugar is better for them?
9. In these days of terrorist threats, how do you protect your health for the long term in the event of a nuclear attack?

These are important questions. At some point, anyone who depends on a chemical diet to solve their nutritional needs must realize that artificial diets AREN'T healthy in the long run. You know that! If you are diabetic, there are natural diets and alternative sugar substitutes other than aspartame or sucralose available on the market. If your children are hyperactive, research the amount of fake fats in their diets, food colorings and other chemicals they are exposed to, and determine if they are getting enough exercise. If you want to lose weight, how much exercise and rest do you *really* get each day?

What underlying issue may be keeping you from changing your lifestyle to prevent needless suffering from a preventable disease – or an early death?

Back up and start over: how do you perceive taking care of yourself? Your body is a tool, and like any instrument needed to complete a task, you must maintain that tool properly to keep it functioning efficiently. Do all you can do to protect your health by eating a natural, balanced diet beginning NOW. What goes into your body must be used to its fullest potential to secure long term health and wellness.

And read! There is an abundance of information on nutrition and disease in public and university libraries dating as far back in time as you choose to probe. The blend of good nutrition and emotional wellness is an art passed down from generation to generation. The causes of modern diseases are harder to identify today than ever before because of the abundance of chemicals flooding our air, water, and food. As time marches on, much information is forgotten. Let's turn back time, and remember wisdom from the past so the future can be filled with peace and health – and no chemicals.

Step Five: Detoxify Your Body

Just as an oil spill pollutes the ocean killing the sea life within, chemicals within your body pollute you and damage healthy cells. Cleaning your body of toxic foods and environmental poisons is no different than restoring a polluted watercourse. The Detoxification Program is a combination of the finest vitamin supplements from around the world orchestrating the perfect tools to remove environmental and food toxins. Complement the supplements with a whole foods diet as natural as possible, and minimize buying packaged food products with ingredient lists that resemble a chemistry book.

WHAT GOES <u>OUT</u> IS JUST AS IMPORTANT AS WHAT GOES <u>IN</u>! Nutritional diets are critical to long-term health, but when you are polluted with chemical toxins from manufactured metals, inoculations, or food additives, it is important to remove these toxins as quickly and as safely as possible. Removing chemicals from the human body is a two-part process – cleansing from the chemicals permeating your tissues <u>and</u> eating right. <u>Give your body a chance to accept healthy dietary changes by cleansing it first.</u>

Many times, removing toxic foreign chemicals from the body can be as simple as turning your diet around. In the case of my

Grave's Disease, however, it's not always so easy. One of the most common questions I hear is: "How do I remove these chemicals from my body?" This Ten Step Program! Read on...

Step Six: Restore Depleted Nutrients

When you walk into a vitamin store, there are thousands of bottles on the shelf and out of all those choices, how do you know what you really need? The hair analysis specifies exactly which nutrients you are depleted in, and those are the vitamins to buy first for your special needs. Some vitamins are a lower quality these days and may contain toxic metals as fillers and have coatings that are hard for the stomach to digest, so research the various vitamin manufacturers for the best. Here's a good rule-of-thumb: <u>If you have to break your vitamins apart with a hammer, they are not a quality product. Natural supplements should be breakable with a slight snap between your fingers.</u>

Food provides all living things with the basic requirements to furnish energy for daily activities. Just as a machine burns gasoline or coal for fuel, the human body burns food for fuel. It's as simple as that. A machine converts its fuel into other forms of energy; the human body converts food into body energy. So why eat fake foods filled with chemicals instead of food bursting with natural nutrients? Think about this the next time you see someone sipping a diet cola while eating a fake-fat-free chunky bar for lunch. And they wonder why they feel tired all the time and have health problems?

Beware of artificial "diets" and diet programs. Remember this fact: if you lose one pound of weight by starving yourself and eating "fake" foods, you actually lose approximately three-quarters of a pound of fat and one-quarter pound of lean muscle mass. However, if you lose one pound of body weight following a whole foods diet with regular exercise, you actually lose approximately one and one-quarter pounds of fat and gain one-quarter pound of lean muscle. Lose weight by eating natural foods and exercising regularly! There's no such thing as healthy *dieting*. Instead, adopt a healthy *lifestyle*. Balance your life. Purify your internal environment.

After my experience with aspartame, I learned to avoid processed, artificial, counterfeit, sugar-free, fat-free, calorie-free, responsibility-free foods. I only eat *real* food. It's more expensive, but it's healthier! And with the money I save on medical expenses, I'm still ahead.

Here are some tips:

1. Lay out a variety of fresh snacks like popcorn, raw nuts, fruit, and veggies after school or work. My kids love it, and they actually eat it!
2. Snack on raw foods every day. Apples, oranges, and raw nuts in the shell – I don't believe animals (including humans) gain weight from raw, healthy foods.
3. Eat big meals early in the day. At night, your body processes what's left over. Try not to eat heavy food past five or six o'clock in the evening.
4. For an evening snack, pop popcorn in cold-pressed seed oil with a little natural butter and sea-salt, drink a fruit smoothie, or enjoy a cup of herbal tea.

We humans, however, have to be reminded to "graze," as most animals do, on <u>small</u> amounts of natural foods during the day, not eating large portions at one sitting, which the body will store as fat.

Tell me what you eat, and I'll tell you what you are. Eating the right foods goes a long way toward radiant health, toward resisting disease, toward securing proper growth for children, and insuring youthfulness and energetic aging for all.

Step Seven: Exercise And Get Plenty Of Rest

Where you find diet colas, processed foods, televisions and computers, stale air and pollution, you'll find people gaining weight and getting sick, and at younger and younger ages. "Modern" human beings don't move their bodies enough. Exercise alone can keep your weight down, yet exercise shouldn't require you to join a fancy health spa and dedicate a half a day to an exercise program. Exercise means:

1. Walking or bicycling instead of taking the car
2. Climbing the stairs instead of riding the elevator
3. Walking the dog after work rather than sitting in front of the television

Children are running, jumping and playing less and less as today's society becomes more stressful and technological.

So, exercise daily. Movement keeps the blood flowing. Blood carries nutrients and oxygen to the entire body, delivering life to every cell. The lymph system can move toxins out of your body. Bodies need to <u>keep moving</u>!

A study from Brown University, USA discovered that 2,500 people who lost an average of sixty pounds and kept it off for a year exercised approximately one hour a day. Another study to complement the Brown Study found that short bouts of exercise throughout the day were as effective as one long period in maintaining weight loss. And eating natural foods as opposed to fake foods with no nutrient value is rudimentary to a healthy exercise program.

And sleep! Sleep is nature's way of putting yourself at rest while the body's immune system comes in to "clean up" like the night-shift cleaning crew. Scientists have determined that after 5:00 P.M. the body is ready to stop eating and start processing what it was fed during the day. It can't do this with a late night meal nor without the body shutting down to rest through sleep. While you are asleep, the body works to repair, cleanse, eliminate all the "leftovers," and strengthen the body organs and organ systems in preparation for the next day. For example, it has been determined that at 1:00 A.M., the liver begins its daily repair and restoration. Each body organ and its supportive body systems take a turn, if you will, so that the immune system can focus on one specific organ at a time. It takes approximately two hours for each organ to be dealt with. If you are not asleep, and even worse, if you are eating at this time, the body can't efficiently do what it needs to do. So you wake up tired, your organs are not rejuvenated, and you may not have eliminated excess body weight, toxins, or water weight. Your body may now be out of balance and will take care of this dilemma the following night. And the cycle begins again.

Step Eight: Eat 75% Raw Foods At Every Meal

Eat *raw*. If there's only time to grab quick food, keep lots of fresh vegetables, natural dry cheeses, whole-grain crackers, pickles, natural yogurts, tofu, fruits and nuts, water and fresh juice on hand. You may have to shop more often because the "real stuff" spoils more quickly, but that's because it's loaded with enzymes and live nutrients - nutrients that actually feed your cells what they require and deliver energy to your living tissues. Raw, lightly steamed, natural, and fresh! All parts of a nutritious quick meal. Plus, eat all you want. It's *hard* to gain weight eating only natural foods. (Note: Don't over-do high-fat natural foods, either, such as shelled nuts. Be balanced in everything you do!)

> Think of your food plate as a "pie" – *no, NOT an apple pie.* Seventy-five percent of that pie should be raw or steamed every meal. These "fundamental" foods provide all the digestive enzymes the body needs, as well as the vitamins and minerals required to trigger the digestive chain reaction.

Basic nutrition doesn't need to be as complicated as food manufacturers and shrewd marketing departments make it out to be today. Remember that fat-free this and sugar-free that and all the modern-day food fads and diet crazes are really nothing but advertising campaigns. Most manufactured foods are filled with toxic fillers and preservatives and have lost their nutrient content, even though the manufacturers claim to have "enriched" the foods by putting manmade artificial, hard-to-absorb vitamins back in before packaging. The required daily amounts of natural vitamins and minerals, amino acids, necessary sugars and fats, and proteins the body demands for fuel cannot be obtained through any source other than raw foods and natural supplements. Don't fool yourself. <u>You're body will know</u>.

Natural foods supply the fuel needed to stay healthy, to keep your body moving, and to stay mentally alert. All food passes through the same set of reactions, whether it's fast food or a raw carrot. What is **in** that food is the issue. Always try to eat 75% foods rich in natural nutrients instead of chemical fillers and toxic by-products.

The natural ability your human body possesses is no less a miracle to select substances from the foods you eat required to build flesh and blood, bones and teeth, and to regulate the countless processes driving respiration, circulation, metabolism, and digestion. Give your body what it needs to stay healthy - not sugar-free, fat-free, fake food chemicals, but 75% of each meal should be fresh, raw food bursting with nutrients.

Step Nine: Drink Water, Water, Water

Water is important in keeping the body strong. Approximately two-thirds of the adult human body is water - <u>salt</u> water. Humans drink fresh water, but we are actually saline. Simply taste a tear or a bead of sweat for its salt content. This is one reason why humans need to drink ample fresh water every day. It keeps the body's salt concentrations low, easing stress on the kidneys and cardiovascular pathways. Plus, the average adult eliminates approximately eight cups of water a day by sweating, urinating, crying and salivating. It is essential to replace what is lost. Drinking lots of water and sweating during exercise helps eliminate toxins, too. And one thing's for sure, if you've been drinking diet colas or iced tea with Equal all day every day, you have NOT been giving your body enough water. And if you are exposed to environmental toxins or radiation, having your body saturated with water will help eliminate those toxins more quickly and more efficiently. So get into the habit of walking around with a bottle of water - all day long. You'll have more energy, feel better and feel full, and flush out toxins quickly.

Chief Oren Lyons of the Onondaga American Indian tribe stated in the book <u>Wisdomkeepers</u>, "One of the Natural Laws is that you've got to keep things pure. Especially the water. Keeping the water pure is one of the first laws of life. If you destroy the water, you destroy life."

Step Ten: Get Control Of Your Life

You must not neglect the fact that healing from a disease or illness takes faith, personal strength, and perseverance. A book I keep close to my side is <u>The Four Agreements</u> by Don Miguel Ruiz. Born into a family of natural healers and raised in rural Mexico, Ruiz was mentored by his mother, a healer, and his grandfather, a native shaman. For more than a decade, he has taught the ancient Toltec traditions, blending ancient wisdom with modern-day personal awareness. I respect Ruiz's work and I practice "The Four Agreements" myself to stay balanced within my daily life. I pass these on to you, because to resist disease requires emotional and spiritual discipline.

Be impeccable with your word. As Ruiz writes, *speak with integrity.* Say only what you mean. Avoid using the word to speak against yourself or to gossip about others. Use the power of your word in the direction of truth and love.

Don't take anything personally. What others say and do is a projection of their own reality. When you are immune to the opinions and actions of others, you won't be the victim of needless suffering. (Many times, it's not about you.)

Don't make assumptions. Find the courage to ask questions and to expect what you really want. Communicate with others as clearly as you can to avoid misunderstandings, sadness, and drama. With just this one agreement, you can completely transform your life.

Always do your best. Your best is going to change from moment to moment; it will be different when you are healthy as opposed to sick. Under any circumstances, simply do your best, and you will avoid judgment, self-abuse, and regret.

As you recover from any chemical poisoning, your entire life will change as a result. You may experience a refreshed emotional outlook as a positive side effect of your lifestyle changes. I designed this Ten Step Program to improve and protect your health and the health of those you love. Removing toxins and manmade chemicals from your life is merely the first step to a complete disease recovery. As you experience affirmative physical changes, may you also begin a journey of self-empowerment and lifelong health.

CHAPTER 6

Dying To Be Thin – Obesity and Diet Sweeteners

Becoming overweight doesn't happen overnight. Day by day and week by week, we eat or drink a little more than our bodies can use for daily energy, growth and physical activity. No matter what the food or beverage is—sugar-free, fat-free or not—the unnecessary calories get stored as fat. Over time, the stored fat accumulates and your weight increases. More energy is coming in than going out.

Do Diet Sweeteners Really Help You Lose Weight, or Do You Eat More and Gain Weight in the Long Run?

According to researchers, there is no clear-cut evidence that sugar substitutes help people lose weight. <u>These days, more and more data suggests that these chemical sweeteners may actually stimulate appetite.</u>

Can Diet Sweeteners Actually Make You Fat?

Yes, because they trick your body and don't feed it what it needs. You <u>stay</u> hungry, so you eat more. Chemical diets are unnatural, and when the body is hungry, it wants to be fed—not chemicals, but whole foods with natural vitamins and nutrients to fuel it.

Fake foods are what I refer to as "prosthetic foods" because a prosthesis looks like the real thing, such as a false tooth, but there is nothing inside of it—it's not real. So it is with fake foods. <u>They may look like real food and taste like real food, but there is nothing inside to feed your body.</u>

Several things happen when the body is fed diet chemicals:

1. It begins to hoard whatever "real" food it receives in the form of fat, because it thinks it's starving and stores food for later use.

2. Artificial food chemicals penetrate the brain and get stuck there, acting "out of control" once inside. They are toxic to the brain, and they upset the normal function of the pineal gland, the hypothalamus and the nerve centers, sending scrambled signals to the body organs. Illness, hormone imbalances and weight gain can result.

3. They stimulate the hunger sensation but do not satisfy your appetite. So, you remain hungry, and <u>you eat more.</u>

Listen To Your Elders: Miriam is my mom. A Rhodes scholar, Miriam is a sharp 81-year-old woman. She was raised during the American Depression of the 1920s, grew up in a small town outside Atlanta, Georgia and lived through the sugar rations of World War II. She became a gourmet cook in her married life, always eating fresh foods and serving our family gourmet, homemade dishes every day. Now a widow, Mom sold her home and moved into an assisted living center after Daddy died. The "institutional" food is unsatisfying compared to what she was used to eating all her life, and she has had a difficult time enjoying her meals. Plus, a petite woman, she has gained weight (while eating less) for the first time in her life as a result of the processed flours and sugars, and canned or frozen meals.

Miriam tells the story of how her assisted living center always serves ice cream or frozen sherbet after each meal, and she usually chooses the ice cream cup. One night, the kitchen ran out of ice cream and served everyone frozen sherbet—sugar-free sherbet. They didn't tell the residents it was sugar-free, but Mom knew immediately. "I knew it was diet because it didn't taste like real sherbet, but what made the biggest impression on me was after I finished eating it, I wasn't satisfied. I felt as if I had not eaten a cupful of sherbet at all, and I could have eaten another one just to feel satisfied. That's the problem with these diet products these days—they don't do anything for you—so you want to eat more just to feel full."

Are You Hungry All the Time? Science Shows Diet Sweeteners Increase Hunger

Most people agree with Miriam: they don't feel satisfied after eating a sugar-free snack or meal. Many scientific studies show the physical reasons why you don't feel full.

> **It's Not Nice To Fool Mother Nature**
> A sweet taste triggers your brain to expect calories and
> carbohydrates (incoming sugar). When you fake out your
> body, and nutrients aren't delivered, the body activates a
> "hunger response," which creates a constant need for food.

Besides affecting insulin, serotonin and your body's hunger
response, chemical sweeteners also increase cravings *in yet
another way* by altering your blood sugar. This can be dangerous
to people with diabetes or epilepsy and can cause fluid retention,
giving the body a puffy and bloated appearance, and it increases
cellulite, too.

Tordoff and Friedman have shown that test animals have
the urge to eat more food up to ninety minutes after ingesting
artificial sweeteners. They documented that when blood levels
for insulin production were normal (high levels of insulin are
believed to be the cause of hunger), the animals that were fed
chemical sweeteners consumed more food than the ones who did
not eat artificial sweeteners.

Science continues to support the phenomenon of appetite
stimulation. Blundel and Hill documented that "most artificial
sweeteners enhance appetite and increase short-term food
intake." They reported: "After ingestion of aspartame, the
volunteers were left with a residual hunger compared to what
they reported after eating glucose (sugar). This lingering hunger
leads to increased food consumption." *To me, this proves the brain
retains the urge to eat when the taste buds are stimulated without
"real" nutrients having actually entered the body.*

Those extra calories you save with that diet cola won't make
much difference if you eat chocolate chip cookies three hours
later because you're hungry. If constantly using diet sweeteners is

actually increasing your appetite, why use them? <u>Common sense tells me that proper diet and exercise are more beneficial in losing body fat and maintaining your weight.</u> Even if you believe that artificial sweeteners help your dieting, is this worth risking your health?

Hunger May Simply Be Thirst—For Water, Not Diet Sodas

Drinking water—not diet colas—can often satisfy that hunger according to Dr. F. Batmanghelidj, M.D. In his book <u>Your Body's Many Cries for Water</u>, he writes, *"Many persons confuse their thirst with hunger.* Thinking they have consumed enough 'water' from their soda, they assume they are hungry and begin to eat more than their body needs for food. In due time, dehydration will cause a gradual gain in weight from overeating as a direct result of confusion of thirst and hunger sensations."

> "It is primitive and simplistic thinking that one could easily lace water with all sorts of pleasure-enhancing chemicals and substitute these fluids for the natural and clean water that the human body needs. Some of these chemicals, caffeine, aspartame, saccharin and alcohol, through their constant lopsided effect on the brain ... [program] the body chemistry with results opposite to the body's natural design."
> - Dr. F. Batmanghelidj, M.D.

Ellington Darden, PhD, states in his book, "A Flat Stomach ASAP," that super hydration, sipping large amounts of water each day, is an important dietary guideline.

So, the next time you think you want a "sugar-free snack," drink a glass of water—not a diet cola—and see if your hunger goes away!

The Right Type of Carbs For Weight Loss

Modern consumers have been misinformed about what carbs really are, and typically eat the wrong types of carbohydrates while avoiding the right ones. <u>So, what ARE the right carbohydrates, anyway?</u>

There are two types of carbohydrates:

1. <u>Complex carbs:</u> "*The Good Guys*"—made in nature, disaccharides and polysaccharides (natural sugars). Complex carbs are found in vegetables, greens and fruits.
2. <u>Simple carbs:</u> "*The Bad Guys*"—manmade, monosaccharide (simple sugars and artificial sweeteners). Simple carbs are found in potatoes, corn, refined grains and grain products, refined pasta, processed foods, baked goods, refined sugar and artificial sweeteners.

What do carbohydrates have to do with weight gain and artificial sweeteners? Just about everything! Complex carbs (natural sugars) are bulky and do not pass through the intestinal wall into the bloodstream. This means little or no weight gain or increase in body fat if food portions are regulated. That's why you need to eat your greens, like Mother told you to!

Simple carbs (manmade sugars) pass through the intestinal wall into the bloodstream. This means weight gain, increased fat and elevated blood sugar that can lead to diabetes. We all should eat fruit and cheese for dessert like our Europeans ancestors used to do, instead of eating our modern sugary treats.

Carbohydrates are the most abundant source of energy found in nature. They are products of plant photosynthesis, which provide the plant's fuel for life in the form of sugar. We are eating the plant's energy, which in turn becomes our own energy. When we eat the right kind of carbs, we are providing our bodies

138

with fuel so we can perform daily activities from thinking to walking up a flight of stairs. *If you are eating a balanced diet with reasonably-sized portions, carbohydrates should not cause weight gain*. But these days we are victims of the "fear of carbs and sugar" fad, and the artificial sweetener manufacturers are taking advantage of this with a marketing frenzy.

Perhaps the manufacturers of Splenda – a simple carbohydrate - are overly optimistic to assume the chemicals implanted in their fake sugar molecules absolutely cannot penetrate the intestinal wall into your bloodstream. Scientists have already proven aspartame <u>does</u> transport throughout your blood and into your brain, resulting in weight gain and increased body fat.

Does Sucralose Cause Weight Gain?

It's too soon to prove sucralose will cause the same weight gain reaction as aspartame has over the past twenty years, but sucralose is a *simple carb* made with chlorine that passes through your liver, just like all foods, and the digestion process begins.

The manufacturers of Splenda claim sucralose passes through the body unabsorbed. They also claim sucralose doesn't react with the body's natural processes, and is not broken down *at all*. But, I do not agree that sucralose passes through the body as an unabsorbed simple carb. The research is beginning to reflect my concern.

With today's weight-conscious society, fewer calories with every meal seem to be the logical answer. But a closer look in the mirror may prove recent statistics are correct: diet sweeteners, while decreasing calories, do not control your weight over a long period of time.

Natural Foods Are Naturally Sweet

Hats off to Kashi® and Cascadian Farms®, two natural food companies that produce whole grain, naturally "low-carb" products. Sitting in front of me is a box of Kashi's Heart to Heart® organic honey-nut-O's cereal. This cereal is a model of what real food should be, especially for growing children. There are <u>no</u> artificial sugars, <u>no</u> hydrogenized fats or oils, and <u>no</u> processed grains or unnatural preservatives.

These products are sweetened with naturally milled organic sugar, organic honey, organic molasses, organic oat flour, barley flour, and organic ground almonds. The only "preservative" is vitamin E, added for freshness. And because this is *real food,* you'll feel full after <u>one</u> bowl. I should know – I just finished one!

What amazed me was, I didn't need to sprinkle sugar or an artificial sweetener on this natural cereal because <u>it already tasted sweet</u>. This shows me that many <u>over-processed foods have little taste, so they require artificial chemicals and sweeteners to restore their original flavor.</u>

So, for all the moms, dads, and nannies out there: the next time you put the "honey nut cereal" in a snack baggie for the kids, choose these brands instead of the "other" ones full of fake chemical fillers and little nutrition. You'll notice an improvement in your children's behavior and their desire to snack.

The Epidemic Of Obesity

<u>The percentage of overweight children has tripled in the past two decades</u>, and the <u>percentage of obese adults has doubled</u>. Even when we factor in bad health habits and poor lifestyle choices, we must acknowledge this weight gain coincides with

the introduction of NutraSweet twenty years ago. *Coincidence?* I don't believe in coincidence, and I strongly believe aspartame and diet sweetener use are directly related to weight gain. Over twenty years ago, independent researchers warned us that aspartame would cause weight gain—*and look at us now.*

Obesity is increasing worldwide and is set to become the world's biggest health problem. Recent reports suggest that it may soon overtake cigarette smoking as a serious health risk. Nearly two-thirds of adults in the United States are overweight, and 30.5 percent are obese, according to data from the 1999-2000 National Health and Nutrition Examination Survey (NHANES). In the UK, nearly two-thirds of men and over half of all women are now overweight—and one in five are obese. At this rate, by 2010 at least one in four adults will be obese. According to data compiled by the International Obesity Task Force (IOTF), England and Scotland have some of the highest levels of obesity in Europe.

The worldwide increase is also spreading to areas of developing countries where there is recent access to the Westernized over-processed diet and technology.

Obesity poses serious health risks such as diabetes, heart disease, cancer and high blood pressure, to name a few. *All of these chronic diseases can be positively altered through proper dietary changes of whole foods <u>without</u> fake sugars or fake fats, so take heart.*

The High Price Of Obesity Includes:
1. Type II diabetes
2. Heart disease
3. Certain cancers (uterine, breast, colorectal, kidney and gallbladder)
4. Stroke
5. Back and joint pain
6. Osteoarthritis
7. Infertility
8. Sleep apnea and other breathing problems
9. Depression
10. Snoring and difficulty sleeping
11. Hypertension
12. Gallbladder disease
13. Osteoarthritis (degeneration of cartilage and bone of joints)
14. High blood cholesterol
15. Complications of pregnancy
16. Menstrual irregularities
17. Hirsute (presence of excess body and facial hair)
18. Stress incontinence (urine leakage caused by weak pelvic-floor muscles)
19. Psychological disorders such as depression
20. Increased surgical risk

Portions DO Matter

The size of your meals DOES matter. <u>Modern consumers, especially children, have no idea how to eat normally</u>. The average consumer eats almost twice the portions of food as twenty years ago. The marketing of artificial sweeteners has been a huge contributing factor to a change in the way people look at their meals. Jean Weininger from the San Francisco Chronicle, USA, writes, "Studies have shown that people who use artificial sweeteners don't necessarily reduce their consumption of sugar—

or their total calorie intake. Having a diet soda makes it okay to eat a double cheeseburger and a chocolate mousse pie."

Instead of loading up on diet products, **try cutting your portions of real food in half.** Dr. Kristine Clark, RD, director of sports nutrition, Pennsylvania State University suggests: "Eat what you want, but eat half. Leave food on your plate—there is no such thing as a 'Clean Plate Club!'" She emphasizes more physical activity on a daily basis along with modifying the portions of your foods and beverages. "This should break the cycle of weight gain," she says.

Super-Size It!

A single twenty-ounce bottle of soda is actually 2 1/2 servings. In America, muffins are the size of small cakes. "Care for a large order of French fries? It's just a few cents more to super-size that order." That's a third of the total calories you should eat in one day! But do people resist the fries? Not usually. They order a large diet cola to justify the difference!

According to a new study by the American Centers for Disease Control and Prevention, women are eating 300 more calories a day and men 168 more calories than twenty years ago. As any nutritionist will tell you, all it takes is one hundred extra calories a day to gain ten pounds a year. To work off those one hundred calories, you must walk twenty-five minutes every day.

In Sting's first book, "Broken Music," he writes about the first time he came to New York City. On a limited budget, he ordered a salad thinking this would be mere rabbit food, yet it was all he could afford. When the salad arrived at his table he was amazed at how large the portion was, and commented in his book that one of the first impressions he had about America was how much food we ate and how much larger the portions were compared to Europeans'.

Many experts feel Americans overeat because much of the food that makes up their modern diet is inexpensive, dense with the taste of "fat" calories, and highly processed, so again, <u>the food isn't satisfying, so we eat more to try to feel full</u>.

How To Control Your Portions

Accurately estimating food portions can be difficult if you are dieting or hungry. This chart makes measuring simple and helps you estimate your portions correctly.

Food Portions:

1. One teaspoon (5 ml)
    - about the size of the top half of your thumb
2. One ounce (28 g)
    - approximately a one-inch cube of cheese
    - volume of four stacked dice
    - slice of cheese is about the size of a 3 1/2-inch computer disk
    - one handful (palm) of nuts
3. Two ounces (57 g)
    - one small chicken leg or thigh
    - 1/2 cup of cottage cheese or tuna
4. Three ounces (85 g) (meat exchanges)
    - serving of meat is about the size of a deck of playing cards
    - 1/2 of whole chicken breast
    - one medium pork chop
    - one small hamburger
    - unbreaded fish fillet
5. 1/2 cup (118 ml)
    - fruit or vegetables can fit in the palm of your hand
    - about the volume of a tennis ball

6. 1 cup (236 ml)
    - about the size of a woman's fist
    - breakfast cereal goes halfway up the side of a
      standard cereal bowl
    - broccoli is about the size of a light bulb
7. One medium apple = a tennis ball

If you were on a budget and taking the kids out for a quick bite after a long day at work, which fast-food restaurant would you choose?

1. *Restaurant A* serves a 2.8-ounce hamburger with a 2.4-ounce bag of fries, and a 6.5-fluid-ounce regular cola
2. *Restaurant B* serves a 4.3-ounce burger with cheese, a 7-ounce carton of fries, and a 16-fluid-ounce diet cola

Restaurant A represents the common take-out meal in <u>1954</u>. Total caloric intake was 491 calories (including the cola), and no neurotoxins or carcinogens were in the drink. *Restaurant B* is the typical carryout in <u>2004</u>. Super-size it for a total of 1,000 calories (cola included), and people seem to justify the larger portions by drinking "diet."

"Super-sizing is a public health issue of the highest priority," said Harvard University's Dr. George Blackburn, a professor of nutrition and surgery. Super-sizing has become so controversial these days, McDonald's, the corporation that popularized the "super-size" concept, announced it was discontinuing its 42-ounce "super-size" soda as well as its seven-ounce "super-size" order of fries at all 13,000 U.S. stores as part of a healthy lifestyle initiative.

What Are We Teaching Our Younger Generation?

Some of the most disturbing weight statistics concern children. Results from the 1999-2000 NHANES Survey, using measured heights and weights, indicate that an estimated fifteen percent of children and adolescents aged six to nineteen years are overweight. This represents a four percent increase from the overweight estimates of eleven percent obtained from NHANES III from 1988 to 1994.

No one can say with certainty whether one cause of childhood obesity outweighs another, but considerable blame can be placed on the fact that kids don't get enough proper nutrition, they sit more, and consume more and more diet products daily.

School Vending Machines: Ditch The Fizz!

Children are encouraged to consume junk food at schools where the influences of fast food and soft drinks are prominent. The marketers of flavor, not nutrition, influence the food and drinks sold in schools.

There is a growing movement against soft drinks in public and private schools. School programs discouraging the sale of carbonated drinks appear to reduce obesity among children. A British study in London showed that reducing young students' intake of sweetened carbonated beverages reduced obesity among the students. A one-year "ditch the fizz" campaign discouraged both sweetened and diet soft drinks among elementary school children. The results showed a decrease in the percentage of children who were overweight or obese. The improvement occurred after the reduction of less than a can of soda a day. Apparently, such programs are working. According to the study, a high intake of carbonated drinks contributed to childhood obesity.

Of course, representatives of the soft drink industry contest these results, claiming carbonated drinks provide only a fraction of children's daily calories, and that they should not be blamed for the childhood obesity epidemic.

In Florida, USA, the Governor's Task Force on Obesity stopped short of admitting soda machines can make kids fat. They suggested a variety of remedies to the state's obesity epidemic—less TV, more exercise in schools—but unfortunately they did not recommend the removal of soda or snack machines from pubic campuses, rationalizing, "The machines often offer milk and other alternatives to carbonated drinks." (Can we trust children to make good choices—after all, they are *children!*)

School vending machines raise considerable cash, funds that many high schools use to support athletic and other extra-curricular activities. Most school principals support the idea of choice and don't want to eliminate the "cash cow" of colas.

Most US state laws protect the sale of carbonated beverages on campuses if fruit juice is also sold. But many districts around the country are trying to get control of the situation in an effort to improve their students' nutrition. In Broward County, Florida, the school board's policy permits vending machine sales for only one hour after the close of the last lunch period.

Corporate Marketing Myths

Do people use artificial sweeteners in foods and beverages even when they are not dieting? Yes, because the biggest myth of all is that food with sugar will make you fat, and diet products will keep you thin, whether you are on a diet or not. Myth #1: Eat all the sugar-free products you want without penalty. Myth #2: Sugar is unhealthy and artificial sweeteners are part of a healthy lifestyle.

More myths:

Myth: As part of a sensible weight-control program, artificial sweeteners can help consumers reduce calories and make it easier to lose weight.

Myth: Artificial sweeteners and diet products provide weight-conscious people with a greater variety of healthy food and beverage choices.

Myth: The ultimate success of any weight-loss program depends on a particular product—not on the responsibility of the individual.

Myth: Human and animal evidence supports complete artificial sweetener safety.

Myth: The majority of health professionals push diet products as beneficial.

Myth: Artificial sweeteners have nothing to do with the rise in degenerative diseases such as ADHD, autism, MS and Parkinson's.

Don't Worry—You Can Make Lifestyle Changes Gradually

Try these suggestions:

1. In restaurants, share entrees or ask the waiter to put half the entree in a doggie bag before you even touch it.
2. Order lunch-sized portions. Many restaurants serve 4 to 6 ounces of meat at lunch, as compared to 8 to 10 ounces at dinner.
3. At home, use smaller plates and bowls. It will look as if you're eating more.
4. Check food labels for serving size. Eat one serving only.
5. Actually measure labeled servings to see their sizes.
6. Drink water when you're hungry for a snack.
7. Instead of drinking soda (regular or diet), drink water (add a squirt of lemon or lime for flavor).

8. Buy smaller packages of candy, popcorn and snacks, or better yet seek out healthy alternatives like raw vegetables, nuts and seeds, fruit, cheese and hardboiled eggs.
9. Do not eat or drink diet products with any meal.
10. As you gradually reduce fake foods and artificial sweeteners in your daily meals, replacing them with whole, nutritious foods, your body will feel satisfied. It is only when you give your body plenty of the real food nutrients it needs and maintain a healthy level of activity that you will be able to eat until you feel full without gaining weight and without feeling hungry.

Don't be discouraged. You can change your lifestyle, not with trendy chemical diets, but with the tried and true methods our bodies recognize and celebrate: whole, natural foods and moderate exercise. Ditch the fizz, drop the fake foods, and your body will respond with vibrant health!

CHAPTER 7

Artificial Sweetener Case Histories

True stories have a way of grabbing our attention – especially when we humans share the same frailties of a flesh-and-blood body and strive to avoid pain and disease. We listen to others so we can avoid their mistakes as well as share in their triumphs.

These are actual experiences of people who suffered from debilitating health problems caused by artificial sweeteners – aspartame, sucralose, and sweetener blends. No "scientific proof" here, just a striking similarity in all the case histories: most of the victims dramatically recovered <u>when they simply stopped using artificial sweeteners</u>.

Although in my work I rely heavily on scientific data, I genuinely respect an individual's personal experience since I, too, was once a victim of Grave's Disease caused by aspartame poisoning. (My "fatal" condition disappeared when I got off diet sweeteners.) If you are sick and the doctors are mystified and can't help, assurances of product safety from a manufacturer mean little. But learning from others how to solve a health mystery and escape illness seems valid. *Success* stories have a way of grabbing our attention, too.

Olympic Diver

When I received a phone call from a young man named Justin Dumais, I thought I was talking to an average young man who had just been diagnosed with a mystifying case of Grave's Disease. He had researched his diagnosis on the Internet, and had discovered my website www.sweetpoison.com. As in my own diagnosis of Grave's, Justin was in excellent physical shape at the time of his diagnosis and had no history of health problems – at all – yet suddenly found himself in the doctor's office with a racing heart rate, lethargy, debilitating headaches, restlessness yet chronic fatigue, sleep apathy, moodiness, vertigo, ringing in the ears, blurred vision, and depression.

Justin refused to accept his diagnosis because he had always been in top physical condition. He knew there was a reason for his baffling illness, but no medical professional could help him. They could only recommend destroying his thyroid gland, leaving him dependent on medications to stay alive.

"I want to be a pilot," he told me. "I am trying to get on with The National Guard, and a diagnosis of Grave's Disease will destroy my chances. Can you help me?"

"You bet I can! Let's talk," I replied.

He had been drinking Diet Coke® regularly, but before now, he never considered aspartame as the cause of health problems. Then he read a copy of my book, Sweet Poison, and immediately stopped using anything containing aspartame. Justin didn't drink alcohol, smoke cigarettes, or take any medications, and he worked out every day. This modest young man told me later that he was training for the 2004 Olympics. The 26-year-old athlete and his brother Troy were an Olympic diving team. And now this Olympian was diagnosed with an incurable thyroid disorder, with no known cause or cure, rare in men, and even more rare for a man in his twenties.

Justin trained an average of six to ten hours every day for the Olympic Trials. He was getting progressively more tired every day, and his workouts were becoming a strain. He was feeling unstable when on the high dive, and no longer had the perfect precision he took pride in. What was happening to him, he wanted to know. Why was this disease attacking a young, healthy Olympian? After he read about my similar experience with aspartame, he found his answers!

He began the 10 Step Detoxification Program, removed all aspartame from his diet, weaned himself from his prescribed medication, and after six weeks, his Grave's Disease was gone. His energy had returned within days, and his vertigo and dizziness on the high dive were history. Justin became his old self again, went on to win the Olympic Trials, and was off to Athens to compete in the 2004 Olympics.

Justin overcame a puzzling thyroid disease in time to finish sixth in the 3-meter springboard at the Athens Olympics, and finished third in the 3-meter synchro with his brother Troy in the June 2005 World Championships. "If I'd never found you, Dr. Hull, and figured out that aspartame was making me dizzy and weak," Justin told me, "I would never have been able to dive in Athens. *Aspartame almost cost me the Olympics*."

Justin, like me, never had Grave's Disease – we both had "aspartame disease," a harmful reaction to the toxins in aspartame. Once all aspartame was removed and its toxins gone, Justin's health returned to normal within a few weeks, as was my recovery experience. Justin's doctor remained open-minded to Justin's recovery, and noted in his medical records that his diagnosis was incorrect, and was not "Grave's." Now Justin's dream to be a pilot could be granted, and in the summer of 2005, Justin retired from diving to fly for the National Guard.

Completely healthy and aspartame-free, Justin cured an incurable disease he never really had. Aspartame almost cost this athlete his Olympic medals and a career as a pilot. Thanks to his courage and his independent thinking, Justin Dumais proved to himself, other Olympians, and to the National Guard that he never had "Grave's Disease" – merely a bad case of aspartame poisoning.

Type II Diabetes

I am an insulin dependent Type II diabetic. I was diagnosed with diabetes in 1989 and my health care team told me that I could use aspartame to satisfy my sweet tooth. Well, to make a long story short, I suffered severe health problems and quit using aspartame completely. My health problems disappeared, except, of course, for the diabetes. Since then I have been using Sweet 'N Low exclusively as my artificial sweetener.

Last fall my husband and I went on a ranch retreat. The first evening I wanted a cup of decaf coffee after dinner. The only artificial sweetener the lodge provided was Splenda. I decided to try it. However, since I had never used it before I was interested to see the effect it would have on my blood sugar so I took a glucose reading. It was 150. I used about 1/2 a packet of Splenda and was pleased with the taste...no bitterness. However, the next morning my fasting glucose was 310-it more than doubled! I can only account for that kind of rise in blood sugar to the Splenda.

I know this is far from scientific evidence that Splenda may not be good for diabetics. I do believe it is not good for me. The only thing I sweeten artificially is my coffee, and I use saccharin. I do not eat artificially "sugar-free" foods. If it is a choice between sugar or aspartame or Splenda, I choose sugar.

More Than A Case Of The Flu

(From my book <u>Sweet Poison:</u> *<u>How The World's Most</u>* *<u>Popular Artificial Sweetener Is Killing Us – My Story</u>*)

December 7, 1987: Patty Crain was a beautiful girl. She enjoyed a normal and healthy life until she mysteriously dropped dead at age twenty-three. Official cause of death: unknown. Patty's mother, Betty Hailand, witnessed the tragedy unfold.

Patty was Betty's adopted daughter. She was the "All-American girl." Out of nowhere, Patty suddenly developed eye problems and experienced blurred vision accompanied by bad headaches. Betty took Patty to have her eyes examined. The doctor found nothing wrong with her eyesight. Patty and Betty were frustrated because they knew something was wrong.

One day after work, Patty returned to her apartment complaining that the blurriness of her vision was intolerable, and she was experiencing unbearable head pain. She progressively got worse through the night and admitted herself to the hospital emergency room early the next morning. The E.R. doctor diagnosed Patty with a common case of the flu. He ordered routine medication for her nausea, prescribed IVs to be administered to her while in the E.R. for severe dehydration (she required three IVs), and sent her home after they had done all they could for her. She was told to drink plenty of liquids, which she did - plenty of diet drinks. She went home and drank countless diet colas to alleviate her dehydration.

Two days later, Patty's health seemed to be returning to normal. Two days after that, Patty was dead on the floor of her apartment, her hands tightly clinched and her tongue sharply bitten. Apparently, she died while home from work around 4:00 PM. Empty diet drink cans were scattered throughout her apartment.

There was no *official* cause for the grand mal seizure that ended Patty's life, but her mother knew what killed her daughter. She maintained Patty died from NutraSweet poisoning.

Betty knew that her daughter was addicted to NutraSweet. Patty regularly drank no fewer than six diet drinks every day and perpetually added more than five packets of Equal to one glass of iced tea.

Betty never stopped believing her daughter's death was connected to her heavy consumption of aspartame. In memory of her daughter's *"cause of death: unknown"* as stated on her death certificate, Betty staunchly battled the NutraSweet Company and fought the suppression of information concerning the dangers connected to this chemical sweetener. As a mother fighting for her child, Betty never gave up the battle to prove she was right.

In 1991, Betty was found shot to death in her Vista, California home. Her assailant broke into the bathroom and shot her while she was in the bathtub. To date, the L.A. police have not apprehended her murderer.

Nutra-Not-So-Sweet

Anna was twenty-two years old but felt like she was ready for her ninety-fifth birthday. Anna started drinking cola when she was thirteen years old. She had a Coke here and there, but felt it was "no biggie." Then at sixteen, Anna began to waitress and free colas were available to her. As a way to keep on the run, she drank more and more soft drinks. Her mother nagged her to get off the colas and onto diet sodas. She was worried Anna was drinking too much sugar. So Anna switched from regular colas to diet colas. She hated the taste at first but it eventually grew on her.

Artificial Sweetener Case Histories

Anna switched jobs and started working at a convenience store where she drank more diet cola. "Hey, they were free," Anna explained. She drank more and more, and would even take some home with her. Then she began to bring home a twelve-pack of diet colas every night.

Anna noticed that her thick, beautiful hair was thinning and falling out at an alarming rate. She worried she was going bald in her twenties. She blamed it on her hair dye for lack of any other logical explanation.

Now, almost twenty-three years old, Anna had been drinking diet colas a long time. It had become an addiction to her. She started drinking a case of diet colas every two days. She felt very sick and her symptoms were the following:

1. Thinning hair: She lost over one-half of her head hair.
2. Weight gain: Anna had normally maintained a constant weight for years, but gained over twenty pounds since she started drinking diet colas.
3. Body aches all over: Anna's joints ached, her neck, her back, *you name it, it hurt!*
4. An ongoing yeast infection: She'd never had a problem with yeast in her life before now.
5. Terrible headaches: Her eyesight worsened, and her head throbbed with a constant ache in the front of her forehead.
6. PMS "from hell" according to Anna: Her cramps were so bad, she couldn't get out of bed at times. All her symptoms of PMS escalated out of control.
7. Bladder infections.
8. Anxiety attacks.
9. Her heart began pounding so badly, she thought she was having a heart attack.
10. Thirsty all the time: She drank that case of diet soda every two days.

11. Depression.
12. Mood swings.
13. Insomnia worsened to the point she would go days without sleep.
14. Tired all the time but couldn't sleep.
15. Anna's face developed a "nasty feeling," dry and rashy. Her complexion flushed after having perfect peaches and cream skin all her life.
16. Restless-leg syndrome: She felt she couldn't hold still when she lay down. She felt the need to run a mile to tire her legs out.
17. Heartburn: "Oh God, yes!" Anna exclaimed. "I'd eat Rolaids like they were candy."

One night Anna was feeling worse than ever. She told her boyfriend what was happening to her, and he suggested she browse the Internet in search of some answers to her mysterious problems. She looked at the back of her diet soda can and the word ASPARTAME jumped out at her. She typed "aspartame" in the search engines and couldn't believe her eyes - her exact symptoms were all listed right there!

Anna immediately stopped drinking all diet drinks with aspartame. The constant throbbing headaches and pain in the front of her head were gone after a mere twelve hours! She was excited to see what else would clear up. One by one over the following weeks, all of Anna's symptoms disappeared once she was off the sweet poison.

Triglycerides And Diet Sweeteners

My physician told me my triglycerides were way too high (over 400), so I tried to alter this number by cutting the sugar and alcohol out of my daily routine. But, I started using diet sweeteners with Splenda because I don't like the taste of aspartame.

I developed intestinal cramping with some random diarrhea, and it didn't help lower my triglycerides at all. I discovered that most of the products with Splenda also contain processed carbs, aspartame, and other chemicals that I can't even pronounce. So, I stopped using the Splenda, began drinking more water, and exercising more.

My triglycerides lowered dramatically.

A Bodybuilder Not Buying Into The Hype Of Diet Sweeteners

Tim is a serious bodybuilder. All the products he purchased for the first year and a half of his career contained aspartame. He started experiencing serious mood swings that increased to the point that he couldn't control himself. Then Tim started a different bodybuilding program without aspartame, and his mood swings disappeared. Upon reading the labels on the protein supplements and meal replacements available, he noticed that some form of artificial sweetener is added to almost all of them. Tim knew how tough it was to drink the supplements without the sweeteners added to make them more pleasing.

He finally found a bodybuilding supplement with fructose, the natural fruit sugar. It was hard for him to find the products he needed to maintain good health, but he continues to advocate the "fresh-raw-real" approach to bodybuilding. The cycle of convenience and dependency is hard to break, but well worth it.

Aspartame Disease

Sharon was a forty-five year old woman from York, Maine who had been drinking diet colas since she was a teenager. Sharon would freely sprinkle Equal® on everything she ate such as pancakes and French toast, and used it in recipes as a sugar substitute. She drank diet drinks every day and used Equal in her coffee every morning. When she read about the dangers of aspartame, she immediately stopped using both NutraSweet and Equal. But Sharon realized she was addicted to these aspartame-containing products when she tried to stop using them cold turkey. She found that she actually craved them, desperately wanting a diet cola about 12:00 or 1:00 in the afternoon.

This especially disturbed Sharon because she could not eat any sugar or fat as a result of gastric bypass surgery she'd had five years earlier.

Sharon suffered with typical aspartame symptoms:

1. Menstrual problems
2. Headaches
3. Poor memory
4. Hair loss
5. Depression
6. Fatigue
7. Joint pain in her right knee
8. Loss of sexual desire

She recently developed a strange cramp in her stomach similar to labor pains. They lasted for several minutes at a time. When she described them to the doctor who performed her gastric surgery, he felt it was an esophagal spasm, something she'd never heard of before.

Sharon also suffered with carpal tunnel syndrome, a condition for which she'd had surgery in hopes of curing the condition. Surgery did nothing. She required constant painkillers with codeine to cope with her pain. She noticed an increase in pain after taking her medication with a diet drink.

When Sharon removed all aspartame from her diet, her daily pain disappeared. She noticed her gastrointestinal problems subsided, and the pain from the carpal tunnel completely disappeared within a few weeks.

"What can I do to help get aspartame off the market?" she asked me. "After all I have gone through, it amazes me this stuff is still being sold."

Parkinson's Disease

In her fifties, Mrs. W held her left hand against her body, using her right hand to keep her palsy from being noticeable. Her involuntary shaking was steadily becoming worse. Her diet was similar to most average Americans, as a considerable portion of it belonged in the garbage can. She never ate seeds or nuts because she was convinced they were "fattening."

Her doctor diagnosed her with Parkinson's Disease. Her nutritionist, however, explained that Parkinson's is a disease of the nerves that can be caused by dietary deficiencies and toxicity. She was asked to eliminate white flour and white sugar products, to eat raw seeds and nuts on a regular basis, and to eliminate all food chemicals from her diet, especially aspartame found in diet drinks. She was asked to supplement her meals with a whole foods diet:

1. An amino acid supplement with at least eight (8) essential amino acid proteins in combination.
2. Three (3) primrose oil capsules per day.
3. Three (3) dolomite tablets both a.m. and p.m.
4. One (1) phosphatidyl choline complex per meal.
5. A quality multivitamin and mineral tablet at breakfast.
6. Two (2) 1,000 mcg. octacosanol tablets (Octacosanol is a waxy substance naturally present in some plant oils and is the primary component of sugar cane extract called policosanol.)
7. Maintain the Detox Program for twelve (12) weeks.

She returned after a couple of weeks to say she felt better than she had in years and to show her left hand no longer shook involuntarily. In fact, her coordination had returned to normal allowing her to resume her hobby of playing golf every day.

Three months later, she called to report her shakes had returned. She admitted she had not taken her supplements for several weeks and had been drinking diet cola every afternoon on her way home from the golf course. The effects of aspartame and the obvious need to restore her health through supplements became apparent when her shakes vanished once again after she stopped using all aspartame and resumed her vitamin program.

My Fibro Is Worse

I have noticed since I started using Splenda products that my Fibromyalgia has gotten worse. My muscles ache more in the mornings, and the bottoms of my feet even hurt when I get out of bed. My lower back aches more, too.

When I stopped drinking my six to seven daily diet colas with Splenda, these symptoms began to decrease. I guess it's because I am drinking more water instead of the Diet Cokes. Boy, I wish I had discovered this information a couple of years ago.

Short But Sweet

Ann constantly drank diet colas. She began to suffer from blinding headaches, spots in her eyes, skin rash, irritable bowel syndrome, a pounding heart, weight gain, dry skin and hair, and severe depression.

She stopped drinking all diet colas, and all of her "mysterious" health symptoms disappeared. She feels younger and has more energy than she did before using diet products.

It is simple. No more aspartame, no more health problems for Ann.

A Woman Who Almost Killed Her Husband

Beth was a qualified medical microbiologist who felt that conventional medicine had been delivering all the wrong answers to her for years. Beth had been feeding her family aspartame with the mistaken belief it was "better" than sugar. "What a dope I was," she confessed. "Much to my eternal gratitude, my sons appear to have suffered no harm as a result of my ignorance, but I almost killed my husband, Arnold."

Here's Beth's story:

Since 1984, Arnold suffered from periodic unexplained blackouts. He was given every possible test - MRI's, CAT scans, DOPPLER scans of his carotid arteries, EKG's, EEG's, and every blood test in the book. One really scary episode resulted in a three-day hospital stay. The hospital and doctors were all convinced he'd had a stroke, despite the fact that he had no risk factors. He showed marked weakness down his right side, slurred speech, and blurred vision. It certainly appeared to be a stroke.

Finally in 1994, he was diagnosed with the seizure disorder, epilepsy. A sleep deprived EEG showed seizure activity. Of course, he'd stayed awake all night by drinking vast quantities of diet colas! The neurologist explained that the "stroke" was something called Todd's Syndrome, where seizures mimic the symptoms of stroke.

Arnold was put on anti-seizure medication beginning with Dilantin, which caused suicidal depression. He was then put on Depakota which almost destroyed his liver (SGOT - 92, SGPT - 219). Then, Tegratol that caused scary personality changes, according to Beth. He became extremely irritable and aggressive, which Beth realized was caused by the effects of the aspartame reacting with the toxic medications. Finally, Arnold was put on Lamictal which appeared to be the best of a bad bunch, and it made him quite lethargic.

The neurologist kept increasing the dosage because of breakthrough seizures. Arnold referred to them as "brain squeezes," which was the only way he could describe the weird sensation he felt.

In the meantime, Beth had read that aspartame was suspected to cause seizures. She never dreamed that was ALL that was causing Arnold's seizures. They decided it was foolhardy to consume something suspected of causing seizures when he already had a seizure disorder. So in October 1996, Arnold gave up all forms of aspartame. He had been drinking several cans of diet soda a day. He also used sugar-free gum and breath mints every day, all day long.

Arnold gradually began decreasing his medication with his doctor's permission. On December 25, 1996 he took his last dose of Lamictal and has not taken any anti-seizure medication since. As of September 1998, he has not had ONE seizure.

Beth was one of the lucky ones. Her own symptoms had been confined to tinnitus and severe headaches, both of which disappeared when she stopped using aspartame.

Arnold and Beth had both put on a lot of weight. After they stopped using products with aspartame, Arnold lost all of his, and Beth had but ten pounds to go. Unfortunately both Beth and Arnold still have severe memory problems as a result of using aspartame. Beth knows that the longer they are off the chemical sweetener, the better their chances of recovery.

Nervous Twitch

A heavy diet soda drinker, Luke noticed he was getting muscle twitches in his eyes, his arms, and even in his chest. The only thing he'd changed in his life was an increase in his consumption of diet colas. So, Luke cut out all diet drinks and began drinking only regular colas. After adding a few pounds, he became disgusted and returned to his diet soda regimen. His muscle twitches came back. He stopped the diet sodas, again, and now refuses to touch anything with aspartame. No more diet drinks - no more twitches.

Childern's Chewable Vitamins With Aspartame

(From my book <u>Sweet Poison: *How The World's Most Popular Artificial Sweetener Is Killing Us – My Story*</u>)

Katrina had been complaining of an earache the very day she went for her three-year check up, Wednesday, January 5, 1994. Odd things had been happening to Katrina, especially her complaints of a stomachache almost daily over the past six to eight weeks.

Katrina had become clumsy, particularly compared to other children her age. Sometimes, she acted blind, literally running into things, and occasionally she fell. At times, she was hyperactive. Her speech became slurred. Her mother, Carmen, wondered if this was typical three-year-old behavior.

Katrina commonly had loose stools, but over the past several months had experienced diarrhea and cramping. The doctor suggested Katrina see a neurologist regarding her periodic "blindness" and falls.

Two days later, her ear pain worsened. She continued falling, once bumping the back of her head quite severely. She kept complaining that her head hurt where her ear was infected.

Carmen called the pediatrician, who prescribed Vantin®, an antibiotic she had used before, and Tylenol® with codeine. She vomited several times that night. The Tylenol never had a chance to get into her system. She couldn't keep anything down. Her parents waited until morning to start the Vantin, and tried a second dose of the Tylenol.

By Saturday, Katrina was lethargic and would not eat anything. Her mother managed to get some sugar-free yogurt down her. Katrina liked yogurt. Carmen hoped she would keep it down. She vomited several times that day. She'd sip on a cold Diet Coke.

The next morning, Katrina was still very lethargic. Her parents decided to take her back to the doctor the next morning if she did not improve that day. At 1:15 pm, Carmen was leaving for work. Katrina had not gotten out of bed for lunch as she normally did. Rather than bothering her sick child, Carmen let her sleep. When she checked on her later, Katrina was lying on her side, motionless. As Carmen got closer, she saw Katrina staring at the wall. She called her name, but Katrina did not respond. She said more loudly, "Katrina?" She still did not move.

She turned Katrina over onto her back. She will never forget what she saw. Her three-year-old daughter lay unconscious, eyes open and glaring, lips and fingernails blue. The right side of her face covered with mucous and saliva from a puddle still pooled on her bed.

Carmen called 911.

Katrina had a seizure while being transported in the ambulance. She had stopped breathing and had to be resuscitated. She was given Valium®, Dilantin®, and Versid®. They performed a CAT scan. After four hours, Katrina was transferred to Riley Children's Hospital at Indiana University where she remained for six weeks. She was on life support for two weeks, in ICU for four weeks.

Katrina continued to have seizures and apnea the first day in the hospital. Doctors performed an MRI, but saw nothing. They did a spinal tap. Nothing. They thought they had her stabilized with anti-convulsants. They extubated her the next day, moving her to the toddler unit.

Her seizures were not typical. Katrina had no jerking of limbs or any physical effects common to seizures. That night, she complained of another bad headache. She could get no relief.

Katrina was put into a Pentobarbital® coma for one week to stop the epileptic seizures. Otherwise, Katrina could die from the damage to her brain by the constant seizing. The doctors wanted her brain wave to be as flat as possible, which they referred to as "burst suppression." During this time, Katrina was on complete life support and a constant EEG monitor. She had an arterial line in her ankle to draw blood hourly to check for blood gases and drug levels. She required a blood transfusion to replace what was being continuously drawn. She had two central lines; one in her neck and one in her groin area. Each central line had two lines leading into it, one for feeding, three for various drugs. Her urine was collected hourly. Katrina was put into isolation as they suspected she was contagious.

For two weeks Katrina was in a coma and on life support. Katrina's family didn't know whether she would live or die. If she did live, could they keep this from happening again? No one could give them any answers.

Katrina soon developed problems with her liver. A liver biopsy was performed. A muscle tissue biopsy was also done. An ophthalmologist was called in to check for a Kayser-Fleischer ring indicating Wilson's Disease. Nothing.

A cytogenetic test was performed, an abdominal ultrasound of her liver and gall bladder. A VER and BSER were performed. The list goes on and on and on. Nothing.

Katrina had an infectious disease specialist diagnose her with non-infectious encephalitis. Her pediatric pulmonologists agreed she had encephalitis, but believed it to be viral. The three spinal taps did not support that opinion, however.

Katrina finally came out of the coma, and was released from the hospital after eight weeks. After spending over $300,000, her parents brought her home. They didn't know what caused her near-death experience or if it would ever occur again. The doctors never determined what really happened.

Katrina was then examined by a gastroenterologist and a neurologist. Katrina's final diagnosis was meningo encephalitis of unknown etiology. No virus found. No bacterial infection discovered. The doctors talked of a possible toxin, but it was never pursued.

Home from the hospital, Katrina was on prescribed anticonvulsants. Her mother did not start her back on her children's vitamins until she weaned her completely from the medication. Seizure-free for over one year, Katrina was given her favorite chewable vitamins. One week later, the same symptoms of her former illness reappeared. Katrina began complaining of stomach pains and diarrhea, and she began stumbling and falling down.

At this time, Carmen was introduced to information concerning aspartame. She began to put two and two together. <u>Aspartame had been in Katrina's vitamins!</u> Carmen took the vitamins away from Katrina, and her symptoms again disappeared.

Artificial Sweetener Case Histories

Three-year old Katrina suffered from:

1. Acute toxicity
2. Lethargy
3. Confusion
4. Impairment of articulation
5. Severe headaches
6. Abdominal pain
7. Vertigo
8. Temporary vision loss
9. Nausea
10. Unsteady gate
11. Unusually high liver enzyme levels

These are symptoms of aspartame toxicity.

Katrina suffered so much. She has a hard life ahead of her. She needs speech therapy. Her behavior is unpredictable. She requires special schooling. Her parents must scrutinize all her meals and snacks for aspartame.

Katrina can never have aspartame again. Yet it is hidden in over 5,000 everyday products. And sometimes it is even found in products not labeled "sugar-free." Her mother has kept her away from all aspartame, and she has never suffered another seizure or related health symptom.

Her life will never be the same. It was an avoidable tragedy.

How would you feel if this were your child?

Perhaps Katrina's heartbreaking story will help another child somewhere – maybe yours – to avoid a lifetime of disability by avoiding artificial chemical sweeteners forever.

CHAPTER 8

Research Studies

The following studies are very long, so I have attempted to translate for the layman the technical jargon in its original form, and included references for each study. (See Appendix References.) I have underlined the research results regarding safety concerns in each of the corporate studies, government reviews, and independent research studies performed outside of corporate influences.

Within this chapter, I have included:

1. Studies on sucralose reviewed by the European Commission
2. Independent studies:
    A. How Sucralose Tastes Sweet
    B. An Independent French Study On Sucralose
    C. A Study From Purdue University On Weight Gain And Chemical Sweetener Consumption
    D. Link Between Kidney Stones And Colas
    E. A Study On DDT Consumption
3. Studies submitted to the American FDA by McNeil Specialties, marketers of Splenda
    A. Diabetic studies in humans

B. Genotoxicity tests
4. Corporate interpretation of McNeil studies submitted to FDA
    A. Sucralose Toxicity
    B. Sucralose Carcinogenicity
    C. Sucralose Teratogenicity
    D. Sucralose Pharmacokinetics
    E. Sucralose Pharmacokinetics and Metabolism
    F. Special Populations
5. A study submitted by Tate & Lyle, the creators of sucralose
6. Toxins in sucralose: a brief explanation
    A. Sulfuryl Chloride
    B. Lithium from Lithium Chloride
7. Splenda Study Submitted To Canadian Government - Trichlorogalactosucrose – Sucralose

Many of the these studies include reports of shrunken thymus glands and spleens, enlarged livers and kidneys, reduced growth weights, infertility, and maternal gastrointestinal disturbances in laboratory rats as a result of varied administered doses of sucralose.

According to the FDA's "Final Rule" report[1]: "Sucralose is weakly mutagenic in a mouse mutation assay." (Showing evidence of mutation.) The FDA also reports other tests submitted as having "inconclusive" results.

According to independent researchers, sucralose is broken down "into small amounts of 1,6-dichlorofructose, a chemical which has not been adequately tested in humans." [2] (See Chapter One.) The following research reports address this concern, particularly the Canadian study at the end of this chapter. It has also been discovered in the research that a compound chemically related to sucrose, 6-chloro-deoxyglucose, is proven to have anti-fertility effects on laboratory animals.

Toxicologist Judith Bellin reviewed some of the sucralose studies on rats that were apparently starved under experimental conditions, and concluded that their growth rate was reduced by as much as one-third without their thymus glands losing significant weight (less than seven percent). Nonetheless, according to the research submitted, the changes in the thymus gland were much more evident in the rats fed sucralose as opposed to those that fasted. While the sucralose animals' growth rates were reduced between seven and twenty percent, their thymuses shrank as much as <u>forty percent</u>.[3]

Note: Contrary to popular belief, the FDA does not perform the product safety studies. The tests are submitted to the FDA by independent researchers and from the corporations themselves for review. The FDA evaluates the results and their rulings are based on the data submitted. Problems were found and approvals were denied when the original sucralose studies were submitted to the Canadian government, the American FDA, and the European Commission.

#1: Studies On Sucralose Reviewed By The European Commission

Research referenced in the European Commission's Health & Consumer Protection Directorate-General's report, *Opinion of the Scientific Committee on Food on sucralose,* adopted by the SCF (Scientific Committee for Food) on September 7, 2000, interestingly shows that all 41 research references submitted to the Committee by Tate & Lyle were unpublished.

The previous SCF evaluations of sucralose are outlined within the EC's report. (See Appendix VIII.) As stated in the report: the SCF first considered an extensive database on sucralose and its hydrolysis products in 1987, and further data submitted in 1988. The Committee's opinion was published in 1989. At that time, the Committee considered sucralose to be **toxicologically unacceptable** due to <u>unresolved questions concerning some of the observed treatment-related effects on body weight, organ weights and hematological parameters</u>. The occurrence of decreased spleen weights, variable thymus weights, increased kidney weights, and the limited clinical chemistry which did not enable liver function to be properly assessed in the original tests submitted to the EC were of great concern to the SCF (Scientific Committee for Food).

According to the European Commission, it was <u>unclear whether the effects observed in laboratory animals might be secondary to being caused by an impalatable taste for sucralose when given in the diet, or if it was due to a direct toxic action of sucralose itself.</u>

The Committee was particularly concerned about the relevance of potential adverse findings relating to the immune system (thymus, spleen, and white blood cell counts). There is also reference in this report to the weak mutagenic activity of one of the hydrolysis products of sucralose, 1,6-DCF. The Committee was, however, satisfied that sucralose had not shown any serious target-directed organ toxicity, and that the sweetener, as such, appeared to pose no carcinogenic or genotoxic potential. At its 70th meeting in December 1989, the Committee outlined the further work it considered necessary to resolve its outstanding questions, and gave their suggestions to the corporations to address.

#2: Independent Studies:

A. How Sucralose Tastes Sweet

According to the research, the drastically increased sweetness of Splenda is due to the structure of the sucralose molecule. <u>Highly intense sweeteners are more hydrophobic in contrast to</u>

more hydrophilic simple sugars, and thus give rise to increased absorption to the taste buds.

According to related research by Deutsch and Hansch in the 1970s (early into the chemical sweetener period), the production of a sweet taste comes from the hydrophobic bonding from one area on a molecule with electronic bonding from another area.[4] Two hydrophobic binding sites necessary for a sweet taste were referred to in their study as A and B. Their findings proved true for all sweet compounds, but interestingly, many other compounds also filled these structure requirements, yet did not have the characteristic of a sweet taste. A later study conducted by Knight and Kier in 1972 recognized the influence of a third site on the molecule, which was hydrophobic *and* bound the sweet compound to the receptor site.[5] This third site was denoted X.

In the case of sucralose, the two chlorine atoms present in the fructose portion of the molecule comprise the hydrophobic X-site, which extends over the entire outer region of the fructose portion of the sucralose molecule. The hydrophobic and hydrophilic regions are situated on opposite ends of the molecule, apparently unaffected by the third chlorine on the C4 of the pyranose ring. The similar structure of sucralose to native sucrose is responsible for its remarkably similar taste to sugar.[6] In laymen's terms: **this is how the chlorine in sucralose tastes sweet.**

According to the producers of Splenda, nevertheless, Wiet and Miller made an opposing assessment of taste.[7] At a sucrose equivalency of eight percent in a buffered (controlled) system, Splenda was perceived as being primarily sweet with slight drying but had sour characteristics compared to sucrose. At a twelve percent sucrose equivalency, sucralose was again perceived to deliver some drying and sour attributes, with a very slight rubbery taste. Such differences in taste assessment indicate that a consumer may find Splenda's taste to resemble natural sucrose, yet not be an exact match.[8]

In conclusion: now we know why Splenda uses chlorine to capture the taste of sugar, but its exact initiation of taste depends on the individual.

B. French Study: No Change In Food Intake Between Sugary Drinks Or Sugar-free Drinks

The following research study was performed on humans to determine the influences of diet colas on food intake and hunger versus the influences of sugary drinks. <u>The conclusion: The diet drinks were less appetizing than the drinks containing sugar.</u> The researchers observed that the food intake was not reduced when using diet sweeteners, and drinking regular beverages induced a positive energy balance as opposed to drinking diet colas.[9]

Objective: To investigate the influence of ingestion of beverages with sucrose or with intense sweeteners on food intake (FI) and on hunger ratings in before and after a month of daily consumption of beverages.

Design: Experimental study. E- drinks = diet drinks, E+ drinks = containing sugar, FI = food intake.

Setting: Department of Physiology, University Hospital, Dijon, France.

Subjects: In all, twelve men and twelve women, aged twenty to twenty-five years of age.

Intervention: Four beverages contained either sucrose (E+:100 g/l, 1672 kJ) or intense sweeteners (E-: null energy content) and were flavored with either orange (O) or raspberry (R). Food Intake (FI) was measured in the lab during two, two-consecutive-day periods, carried out on two successive weeks (session 1). The subjects drank two, one of either E+ or E- beverages on the first day of both weekly periods, according to a balanced randomized design. E+ was paired with zero range for fifty percent of subjects and with R for the other fifty percent. Subjects were then habituated over a four-week period to both beverages, consuming one, l of E+ beverage on odd days and one, l of E- drink on even days. After this period, the measurements of session one were repeated (session two, weeks seven to eight). Finally, FI was measured for two more two-day periods (weeks nine to ten) after the association between flavor and energy content was reversed (session 3).

Results: The E- drinks (diet drinks) were less palatable than the E+ drinks (containing sugar). They observed that FI (food intake) was not reduced in response to a liquid extra caloric load, and there was no change in hunger ratings after the beverages in any of the sessions.

Conclusion: Ingestion of caloric beverages induced a positive energy balance, and the continuous exposure to these beverages over a one-month period did not improve FI adaptation in response to the extra energy provided by the beverages.

C. Purdue Study: Rats Fed Sweetener, Not Sugar, Consume More Calories

Indianapolis — Rats fed artificial sweeteners ate three times the calories of rats given sugar, according to a study suggesting sugar-free foods may play a role in the nation's obesity epidemic. [10]

Purdue University researchers said their rodent findings could help explain why Americans have grown fatter over the past two decades even as U.S. consumption of artificially sweetened sodas and snack foods has soared.

They concluded that artificial sweeteners interfere with people's natural ability to regulate how much they eat by distinguishing between high- and low- calorie sweets.

As part of their study, they fed two groups of rats sweet-flavored liquids for 10 days. One group got only sugar-sweetened liquids, while the other was fed liquids sweetened by both sugar and artificial sweeteners.

After the 10 days, both groups of rats were given a sugary, chocolate-flavored snack and regular rat chow.

Both rat groups ate about the same amount of the chocolate snack. But the rats fed both sugar and artificial sweeteners ate three times the calories of the rat chow than the rats fed only the sugar-sweetened drink.

Susan Swithers, an associate professor of psychological sciences at Purdue, said the findings suggest the rats given the chemically-sweetened drink ate more rat chow because they experienced an inconsistent relationship between sweet taste and calories. That, in turn, could confuse their natural ability to keep track of calories.

"Consuming artificially sweetened products may interfere with one of the automatic processes our bodies use to regulate calorie intake," stated Swithers.

Adam Drewnowski, director of nutritional sciences at the University of Washington in Seattle, said that whatever caused the rats to overeat is unclear and could have been caused by something other than the sugar-free liquid they were fed. He said the rat results have no bearing on human research. [11]

D. Link Between Kidney Stones And Colas

Kidney (urinary) stones are one of the most painful disorders for a humans being and one of the most common disorders of the urinary tract. According to the National Institute of Diabetes and Digestive and Kidney Diseases (NIDDK), more than one million cases of kidney stones were diagnosed in 1985. NIDDK estimates that ten percent of all Americans will have a kidney stone during their lifetime. Several times more men, frequently between the ages of twenty and forty, are affected more than women. Young men are also the heaviest consumers of soft drinks.

Suggesting a link between soft drinks and kidney stones, researchers conducted an intervention trial that involved 1,009 men who had suffered kidney stones and drank at least 5 1/3 ounces of cola per day. One-half the men were asked to refrain from drinking colas, while the others were not.

Over a three-year period, drinkers of Coca-Cola and other cola beverages acidified only with phosphoric acid and who reduced their consumption to less than half their customary levels were one-third less likely to experience a recurrence of kidney stones. Among those who usually drank soft drinks acidified with citric acid (with or without phosphoric acid), drinking less had no effect. While more research needs to be done on the cola-stone connection, the NIDDK includes cola beverages on a list of foods that doctors may advise patients to avoid.

E. DDT Study: Studies On Human and Animal Consumption of Organchlorides (DDT)

This study is an excellent example of the carcinogenic qualities of chlorine-containing compounds to human exposure.

5.2 Human carcinogenicity data

In the Yusho and Yucheng studies, each involving about 2000 cases, humans were exposed to sufficient PCBs and PCDFs to produce health symptoms. Fatal liver disease is 2 to 3 times more frequent than national rates in both participants. In Japan, at a benchmark 22-year follow-up, there was a three-fold excess of liver cancer mortality in men, which was already detectable and even higher at 15 years of follow-up. In Taiwan, at 12 years of follow-up, there was no excess of liver cancer mortality. This difference does not appear to be the result of study design, differences in diagnostic habits, exposure or age at exposure, but may be related to differences in the time of follow-up.[12]

5.3 Animal carcinogenicity data

2,3,7,8-Tetrachlorodibenzofuran (2,3,7,8-TCDF) treatment following a single dose of N-methyl-N-nitro-N'-nitrosoguanidine (MNNG) resulted in an increased incidence of mouse skin papillomas*.[13]

2,3,4,7,8-Pentachlorodibenzofuran (2,3,4,7,8-PeCDF) treatment following a single dose of MNNG resulted in an increased incidence of mouse skin papillomas. 2,3,4,7,8-PeCDF treatment following four weeks' treatment with N-nitrosodiethylamine (NDEA) resulted in an increased incidence of hepatocellular carcinomas and hyperplastic nodules in male rats. Treatment with the same compound after a single dose of NDEA increased the incidence of focal hepatic lesions in female rats. [14]

1,2,3,4,7,8-Hexachlorodibenzofuran (1,2,3,4,7,8-HxCDF) treatment following a single dose of MNNG resulted in an increased incidence of mouse skin papillomas. 1,2,3,4,7,8-HxCDF treatment following four weeks' treatment with NDEA resulted in an increased incidence of hepatocellular carcinomas and hyperplastic nodules in male rats. Treatment with the same compound after a single dose of NDEA increased the incidence of focal hepatic lesions in female rats.

* family of viruses that causes warts and has been implicated as a possible cause of genital cancers

#3: Studies Submitted To The American Fda By Mcneil Specialties, Marketers Of Splenda

A. FDA Rules and Regulations Federal Register Report Vol. 63, No. 64, 16425 d. Diabetic studies in humans (E156, E157, E168, E170, E171) [15]:

Note: These studies were performed and submitted to the FDA by McNeil Nutritionals (the marketers of Splenda) after being questioned by Canadian officials because of three particular issues of concern raised by the FDA review panel:

1. During the course of the FDA's evaluation of the sucralose petition, McNeil submitted additional studies that had been conducted in response to questions and concerns raised by the government reviewing bodies of other countries.
2. In response to an issue raised by the FDA, McNeil submitted a six-month sucralose feeding study in rats with a dietary restriction design to evaluate the toxicological significance of a body weight gain decrement effect observed in sucralose treated rats, When body weight generally decreases in similar case studies, toxicity is noted.
3. In anticipation of the potential wide use of sucralose in persons with diabetes mellitus and to address concerns raised by a diabetic association in Canada, McNeil also performed a series of "requested" clinical studies.

E156 (first series of tests): A single-dose cross-over study (E156) was performed on 13 insulin-dependent (Type I diabetics) and 13 non-insulin dependent diabetics (Type II diabetics) to evaluate the effects of a single dose of sucralose (**1,000 mg**) on short-term glucose homeostasis: future tests submitted were performed using lower doses of sucralose (**100 mg**), yet documentation was submitted using lower dose parameters intended to represent the final results from tests using 1,000 mg

1. Fasting plasma glucose area under the curve (AUC) and fasting serum C-peptide AUC were measured after consumption of a standardized liquid breakfast meal with no mention of fasting after mid-night the previous night of the test,

2. This study showed that neither plasma glucose nor serum C-peptide levels were affected by this single dose administration of sucralose - again with no mention of fasting the night before – if no fasting did take place, serum and glucose levels would not be adversely effected in the same way,

3. From this study, the agency concluded that sucralose did not adversely affect short-tern glycemic control in persons with diabetes mellitus,

4. <u>But note: these studies were not the same-Serum insulin levels measured in study E157.</u>

   E157 (second series of tests): A six-month clinical study (E157) was performed investigating the effect of sucralose (667 mg/d through oral administration) on glucose homeostasis in patients with Type II diabetes, with a decrease in mg from **1,000 mg to 667 mg:**

- Percent concentration of glycosylated hemoglobin (HbA1c) was the primary marker for long-term glycemic control in this study.
- In addition, the following parameters of glucose homeostasis were measured:
    1. Fasting levels of plasma insulin, serum C-peptide, and serum insulin,
    2. Postprandial measures of plasma glucose, serum C-peptide, and serum insulin. (Generally, when serum insulin is measured, the test results are less precise),
    3. These parameters were measured after 0,1,3, and 6 months of treatment.
- The results of this study showed a small but <u>statistically</u>

<u>significant</u> increase in the glycoslyation (long-term blood glucose levels) of hemoglobin (HbA1c).

- This HbA1c effect was observed in the sucralose-treated group <u>at one month of treatment</u>, and did not significantly increase to higher levels throughout the remainder of the study.
- Because of the small patient group sizes in this study, the ultimate clinical significance of the observed HbA1c effect could not be determined. (No reasons were given.)
- <u>However, increases in glycoslyation imply lessening control of diabetes.</u>

Thus, the petitioner performed studies E168 and E170 in an attempt to provide an explanation of the observed HbA1c effect in study E157.

- Because of results observed in diabetic patients treated with sucralose in the previously submitted and evaluated six-month clinical studies, McNeil, themselves, requested in 1995 that the FDA <u>withhold its final decision on the safety of sucralose until that observation could be further investigated</u>. At that time, McNeil initiated additional studies with the main objective of evaluating the effects sucralose would have on glucose homeostasis in patients with diabetes mellitus. These additional tests run by McNeil were also not performed with the same test protocols/parameters previously submitted. Some of the tests were actually not performed on humans, but merely on blood samples within test tubes, yet the <u>results submitted were documented to equate the previous uncertain human diabetic studies</u>.
- The repeated tests submitted were again performed using lower doses of sucralose (**100 mg**), yet submitted so to link the results from tests using **1,000 mg** in the primary

studies.

- There was no mention of fasting after mid-night the previous night of the test.
- This study showed that neither plasma glucose nor serum C-peptide levels were affected by this single dose administration of sucralose, again with no mention of fasting the night before. **If no fasting did take place, serum and glucose levels would not be adversely affected in the same way.**
- *From this study,* the agency concluded that sucralose does not adversely affect short-tern glycemic control in persons with diabetes mellitus.

Note: Serum insulin levels were not measured in this study but were measured in study E157.

E168 (third series of tests): In this study, McNeil performed a series of tests to determine whether the increased HbA1c levels observed in study E157 were an artifact of measurement or a direct effect of sucralose on the rate of hemoglobin glycation: Results from these tests confirmed that in E157, HbA1c (long-term glucose levels) were increased in the sucralose-treated diabetic patients, **the second time the increase in glucose levels were confirmed.**

E157 showed that sucralose had no direct effect on the rate of hemoglobin glycation (blood sugar *decrease* or ionic exchange). This conclusion has never been emphasized.

E170 (fourth series of tests): This study was not performed on humans, rats, or any other animal, but performed in test tubes. Red cell preparations from the blood of diabetic and non-diabetic patients were <u>treated</u> with sucralose (100 mg per liter) – <u>a lower dosage compared to the other tests</u> - to investigate the rate of formation of glycated hemoglobin in the blood.

The results of this study showed:

1. Sucralose did not effect the rate of formation of glycated hemoglobin (a blood sugar decrease).
2. There was no evidence that a physiochemical or other physical influence by sucralose might explain the increased glycation of hemoglobin.

E171 (fifth and final series of tests concerning diabetic reactions): Because studies E168 and E170 did not provide an explanation for the HbA1c effect observed in study E157, study E171 was performed as a repeat of study E157 with, again, "modified" experimental designs resulting in more favorable final results on humans.

1. E171 had **larger patient (human) group sizes and stronger statistical power** (90 percent versus 80 percent in study E157) to detect an effect by sucralose on hemoglycation
2. **A shorter evaluation time was set.** A three-month duration for study E171 (opposed to the six-month observation period for study E157) was deemed adequate because the increased HbA1c levels that were seen at one month of treatment in study E157 did not appear to increase at any of the later time points in the prior study.

In study E171, 136 NIDDM patients (patients with Type II diabetes) were divided into two groups based on their diabetic therapy; 64 were taking insulin and 72 were on OHA's). Each of these two groups were subdivided equally into a sucralose and placebo group. The study was then divided into a screening phase, a testing phase, and a follow-up phase. Glycosylated hemoglobin (HbA1c) was the primary measure of glucose homeostasis. In addition, the secondary parameters, fasting plasma glucose and serum C-peptide, were measured. **Serum insulin levels were not measured in this study, but were measured in E157.**

The FDA concluded from the results of this particular study that sucralose administered at 667 mg/d had no effect on long-term glucose homeostasis (as measured by HbA1c) in patients with NIDDM (Type II). They also concluded that the small but statistically significant decline in glycemic control observed in study E157 within one-month of observations was not a clinically significant effect because the same effect was not duplicated in a repeat study (E171) that had a greater statistical power. Even though the **mg/d** varied from the previous McNeil studies, **no measures of serum insulin levels were measured in the later studies**, and **the duration was of the test had been shortened**, McNeil finally secured FDA approval at 667 mg/d.

The FDA also concluded (based on E171) that as a result of this study, sucralose does not adversely affect glucose homeostasis in patients with diabetes mellitus. (**But no studies within this FDA report were performed specifically on diabetes mellitus, but rather on Type I and Type II specified diabetic parameters.**)

B. FDA Rules and Regulations Federal Register Report Vol. 63, No. 64, 16419, Genotoxicity Testing

The following is a study submitted by McNeil Nutritionals for FDA approval of Splenda based on genotoxicity results of administering sucralose to rats used to predict the carcinogenic potential of sucralose. From the wording in the FDA files, it appears that the short-term testing for the carcinogenic potential of sucralose is inconclusive, and negative responses to sucralose by the rats were observed.

Research Studies

Sucralose and its hydrolysis products were tested in several in vitro and **short-term** in vivo genotoxicity tests:

1. A chromosomal aberration test in cultural human lymphocytes (E012) were **inconclusive.**
2. Sucralose was **weakly mutagenic** in a mouse lymphoma mutation assay (E014).
3. Other assays [**human lumphocytes** (E012)], rat bone marrow (E027) were **inconclusive.**
4. 1,6-DCF was **weakly mutagenic** (E020).
5. Both sucralose and its hydrolysis products **showed weakly genotoxic responses** in some of the genotoxicity tests.

FYI: Despite FDA approval after extensive corporate clinical trials indicating sucralose safety, consumer concern remains high concerning long-term dosage safety. Cyclamate and aspartame were granted FDA approval and successfully reached the market, only to later be implicated as having possible carcinogenic, toxic, and other major side effects. Naturally, consumers of artificial sweeteners would have concern for the safety of a newly developed product. However, the corporations manufacturing and marketing Splenda maintain that FDA approval verifies sucralose safety both after short-term and long-term use. Currently, U.S. Congressional hearings are challenging similar corporate claims for products approved by the FDA such as Teflon® and Merck's popular arthritis drug Vioxx®.

The creators of sucralose, Tate & Lyle, and the marketers of Splenda, McNeil Specialties, claim the results of safety evaluation studies conducted on sucralose have shown it to be a remarkably safe and inert ingredient. McNeil representatives L. Goldsmith and H. Grice have noted that over 100 studies show no signs of carcinogenicity, reproductive toxicology, neurotoxicology, or genetic toxicology as a result of sucralose administration over all clinical study parameters. (But how many of these studies are still unpublished?) Independent research results often differ from the product manufacturers' results.

#4: Corporate Interpretation Of Mcneil Studies Submitted To FDA

The following studies were supervised by Dr. Leslie Goldsmith, Vice President, Safety and Science Affairs, McNeil Nutritionals, reflecting corporate interpretation of the studies McNeil submitted to the FDA for the approval of Splenda containing sucralose: [16]

A. Sucralose Toxicity Tests

Results from over one hundred animal and clinical studies included in this FDA approval process unanimously indicated a lack of risk associated with sucralose intake. Acceptable human intakes across all populations have been pinpointed. The estimated daily intake (EDI) for humans is 1.1mg/kg/day. The intakes acceptable daily intake (ADI) is 16 mg/kg/day. The highest no adverse effects limit (HNEL) is 1500 mg/kg/day.

Sucralose administration to Sprague-Dawley and COBS CD (SD) BR rats, mice, beagle dogs, monkeys, and eventually humans showed no signs of toxicity, carcinogenicity, or other side effects. Studies ranged from single dose administration to eating trials of over two years. Common methods of administration included oral, gavage, and IV intakes. No adverse reactions were observed at intakes up to 16,000 mg/kg/day in mice or 10,000 mg/kg/day in rats—a dosage equivalent to 1,000 pounds of sucrose administered in a single day to a 165-pound adult.

Corporate clinical studies that monitored for chronic toxicity equally resulted in a lack of adverse effects. Acute oral sucralose in-water dosing of male and female COBS CD (SD) BR rats (n=30 per sucralose concentration) and ICI Alderly Park mice (n-10 male, 10 female) resulted in no toxicological effects at four and eight weeks, except for a decrease in food consumption for rats dosed at 5 percent dietary sucralose due to decreased palatiblity. Decreased palatability (rejected the taste) was exclusively observed across several studies involving high-level sucralose administration to rats. [17]

A continuation of the Goldsmith study showed no chronic toxicity in beagle dogs (n=4 male, 4 female) over the course of fifty-two weeks. Comprehensive hematological parameters for toxicity indications included packed cell volume, hematoglobin, mean cell hemoglobin concentration, red blood cell count, mean corpuscular volume, reticulocytes, white blood cell count, alkaline phosphatase level and activity, platlets, prothrombin activity time, alanine amintotransferase, aspartate aminotransferase activity, urea, gluclose, total bilirubin, cholesterol, etc.

Animal studies indicated a lack of neurotoxic effects as a result of sucralose intake. "No morphological or functional signs of neurotoxicity were seen in any study conducted," stated Goldsmith. "Additionally, neither light nor electron system tissues revealed any abnormalities. There was no evidence of clinical or pathological neurotoxicity." Results of a neurotoxicity study performed on sucralose and its two constituent chlorinated monosaccharide hydrolysis products, 1,6-DCG and 4-CG, were compared for their neurotoxicity with a known non-sucralose monosaccharide called 6-CG. 6-CG previously was discovered to have neurotoxic effects in animal studies. Mice (n=30 male, 30 female) and Marmoset monkeys (n=12 male) were treated with sucralose, 1,6-DCG, 4-CG, and 6-CG by gavage at various single dose experiment rations and at various individual concentrations. Evaluation by clinical pathology, light microscopy, and electron microscopy showed an absence of neurotoxicity with sucralose or sucralose hydrolysis product administration, when compared with the 6-CG control.[18]

The potential for sucralose to induce heritable gene mutations was investigated by McNeil representatives in numerous studies on bacterial and mammalian cells and in whole animals. The results of these studies indicated that mutagenicty is not a concern. According to the producers of Splenda, a two-generation rat reproduction study found no evidence of effects from sucralose on male or female mating performance. No effects on reproductive capability were found. Similarly, there were no observed effects on gestation, litter size, or viability of progeny, even at maximum dietary concentrations according to McNeil. Gross, visceral, and skeletal examinations of sacrificed rat offspring showed that sucralose did not affect fetal development.

B. Sucralose Carcinogenicity Tests

Two studies performed by the producers of Splenda demonstrated the lack of toxic or carcinogenic effects due to sucralose product intake. In the first study, CD-1 mice (n=52 male, 52 female) received 0.3%, 1.0%, or 3.0% oral sucralose over 104 weeks. No effects upon survival or carcinogenicity were found. Sucralose administration resulted in no effect upon tumor frequency or type in comparison with controls. Sucralose was determined to not be carcinogenic in CD-1 mice at the maximum tolerated dose of 3 percent.[19]

In the second study, Sprague-Dawley rats were exposed to dietary sucralose concentrations both in utero and up to 104 weeks after parturition.[20] Gavage study toxicity results (n=30 male, 30 female) and carcinogenicity results (n=50 male, 50 female) indicated no effects at dietary concentrations ranging from 0.3 percent – 3 percent, compared with the human sucralose highest-no-adverse-effect level of 1,500 mg/kg/day, estimated daily intake of 1.1 m g/kg/day, and acceptable daily intake of 15 mg/kg/day.[21] A decrease in body weight was noted at 5 percent. <u>This decrease was attributed to decreased food consumption due to decreased palatability. Decreased consumption due to suspect decreased palatability was noted across multiple studies exclusively involving rats.</u> No difference in tumor type or frequency was found between experimental and control groups. There were no ophthalmologic changes found due to sucralose administration. All experimental groups had a decrease in blood glucose level. Sucralose did not adversely affect reproductive or developmental parameters and showed no toxic or carcinogenic effects.

C. Sucralose Teratogenicity Tests

Teratogenic potential of sucralose (its potential and ability to break down) was studied in rats and rabbits during fetal organogenesis. McNeil Specialty research previously indicated the possibility that small amounts of sucralose could cross the human placenta.[22] The effects of this sucralose movement on fetal development were still unknown. Groups of 20 mated rats of 6 - 15 says of gestation and groups of 16 - 18 artificially inseminated rabbits were administered various experimental sucralose concentrations by gavage. Control animals received only the vehicle of administration. At 21 days of gestation, no anomalies related to sucralose were observed in the dams. Fetal and placental weights were comparable to those of the control. **Pregnant female rats showed signs of gastrointestinal distress, due to undigested sucralose.** No adverse affects were observed in the fetuses. The progress of pregnancy and fetal development in rats and mice were unaffected by sucralose up to levels exceeding maternally tolerant levels.

D. Sucralose Pharmacokinetics Tests

Results from numerous studies following sucralose pharmacokinetics confirmed that in humans, approximately 85 percent of ingested sucralose was excreted after intake and approximately **15 percent was absorbed**. Studies with radio-labelled sucralose in rats, dogs, and humans have shown that **sucralose was passively absorbed through the small intestine in limited amounts**. Mean absorption in humans was approximately 15 percent of the ingested dose.

The remainder of the ingested sucralose passed through the digestive system unchanged and was excreted in the feces, with no resulting gastro-intestinal effects. <u>Of the small portion of the initial dose that was absorbed, most was eliminated unchanged via urine, with the majority being excreted within 24-hours after dosage. Total elimination was virtually complete within a few days.</u> Results from rat studies demonstrated that metabolic handling of sucralose was not altered over the course of long-term dosage when compared with short-term dosage. Results from human and animal studies showed that no bioaccumulation was found. (Note: elimination that doesn't take place merely hours after ingestion can be considered bioaccumulation.)

McNeil states: "The relatively small amount of sucralose that is absorbed is distributed to essentially all tissues. There is not active transport of sucralose across the blood-brain barrier to the central nervous system, across the placental barrier, or from the mammary gland into milk." **Although passive movement of sucralose across the placenta does occur**, studies using radiolabelled sucralose in pregnant animals have shown that the levels of sucralose found in the placenta and fetus do not exceed those found in the maternal blood." The equimolar concentrations of labeled sucralose do not accumulate in the developing fetus. <u>The consistency of studies indicating a lack of sucralose toxicity indicates that even if fetal accumulation were found, no toxicity would result.</u>[23]

Doses of radioactive 14C-sucralose by IV and by oral gavage were administered to beagle dogs (n=2 male, 2 female) to study sucralose pharmacokinetics and metabolism. Plasma, urine, and fecal samples were collected and monitored for radioactivity. Beagle urine samples were compared with samples from human males given a single oral dose of 14C-sucralose. Unchanged sucralose was the major component after either oral or IV administration. Significant small amount (2-8 percent of oral dose) of sucralose urinary metabolite glucuronic acid was detected by mass spectrometry. Glucuronic acid metabolite was resistant to hydrolysis. IV administration to dogs resulted mainly in urinary excretion. Oral gavage in dogs resulted mainly in fecal excretion. Fecal excretion accounted for a mean of 65.9 percent of dose during the first 24 hours, increasing to 68.4 percent after five days. Urinary excretion accounted for means of 13.8 percent, 22.3 percent, and 26.5 percent or oral dose after 6, 12, and 24 hours post dosing, respectively, increasing to 27.6 percent after five days. Over the course of five days, the mean total of urinary excretion, fecal excretion, and cage washings was 97.6 percent. The minor metabolite in human urine, glucuronic acid conjugate of sucralose, was co-chromatographed against one of the two minor radioactive components isolated from experimental beagle dog samples, relating this study to sucralose pharmacokinetics and metabolism in man.[24]

E. Another Corporate Example Of A Sucralose Pharmacokinetics And Metabolism Animal Study

John et al. study[25] demonstrated that doses of radioactive 14C-sucralose (20 mg/kg body weight) by tail injection and by oral gavage in isotonic saline were administered to CD-1 mice. Isotonic saline IV sucralose solution was administered via tail injection (5ul/g body weight) (n=4 male, 4 female). Isotonic saline solution (20ul/g body weight) was administered by gavage to three groups of rats: 100 mg/kg body weight (n=4 male, 4 female), 1,500 mg/kg body weight (n=2 male, 2 female), and 3,000 mg/kg-body weight (n=2 male, 2 female). Reactivity in all samples was measured by liquid scintillation analysis. Urine and fecal samples were collected and monitored for radioactivity. The 20 mg/kg IV dose was rapidly excreted, primarily via urine at 80% after five days. The 100, 1,500, and 3,000 mg/kg oral doses resulted in urinary excretions of 23 percent, 15 percent, and 16 percent, respectively, after five days. Comparisons with the IV dose experimental results indicated that 20 – 30 percent of the oral dose was absorbed. Chromatographic urine sample analysis showed that **unchanged sucralose was the main excretory**

form of sucralose in all samples. The minor metabolite in human urine, glucuronic acid conjugate of sucralose (originally identified in the dog) was co-chromatographed against one of the two minor radioactive components found in experimental urine samples. The other minor metabolite was hypothesized to be another glucuronide conjugate. These results indicated that the metabolism of orally dosed sucralose in the mouse is similar to the metabolism of orally dosed sucralose in humans.

The purpose of the Roberts study (corporate submission) was to apply results from previous animal studies and confirm that they hold true for humans.[26] A preliminary and *unpublished* study of three males showed limited absorption, a peak plasma sucralose concentration after two hours of administration, and the absence of carbon from sucralose sources expelled in CO2. In this, study, highly purified radiolabelled 14C-sucralose was monitored for its metabolic and pharmacokinetic activity within a larger cohort.

Two sub-studies comprised the Roberts study. The first was an extension of the preliminary study. Healthy males, mean 39 years, 79 kg weight (n=8) received an oral sucralose dose of 1 mg/kg in water. Blood samples were collected in heparinized tubes immediately before dosing and at 19 proceeding intervals. Administration duration was 72 hours. The second sub-study (n=2 out of the original 8 subjects with higher than average 14C-sucralose excretion) involved an oral dose of 10 mg/kg body weight. Urine samples from subjects involved with both studies were collected prior to dosing and sequentially thereafter for a duration of 120 hours. Fecal material was collected for 120 hours. Concentration of radioactivity was monitored in all biological samples, but the controls received non-radioactive sucralose.

Results from both studies indicated that radioactivity was mainly excreted in the feces over five days, with a mean recovery of 78.3 percent of the oral dose. Urinary excretion for low dose varied between 8.9 and 11.2 percent. The sum excretion by urine and feces over five days averaged 92.8 percent. Results indicated that essentially all recovered sucralose was excreted through the feces and confirmed the lack of sucralose accumulation within the body.

Animal studies <u>performed by McNeil</u> have demonstrated that sucralose is not toxic or teratogenic, has virtually no effect on metabolism, and is rapidly eliminated from the body. Another McNeil clinical study showed that being in the state of pregnancy does not alter sucralose pharmacokinetics or metabolism. Pregnant (n=3) and non-pregnant (n=3) New Zealand White rabbits were given a single oral 10 mg 14C-sucralose/kg dose by syringe in 15 - 20 ml distilled water. Radioactivity was measured by liquid scintillation analysis. Non-pregnant urinary excretion was 8 percent and fecal excretion was 17 percent of the oral dose after 24 hours. Urinary excretion increased to 22.3 percent and fecal excretion increased to 54.7 percent after five days. Pregnant urinary excretion was 9 percent and fecal excretion was 28 percent of the oral dose after 24 hours. Urinary excretion increased to 21.5 percent and fecal excretion increased to 65.2 percent after five days. Remaining 14C-sucralose was found in biliary excretion and in the enterhepatic circulation. These results of the corporate studies on rats indicate that pregnancy does not significantly influence sucralose pharmacokinetcs. [27]

F. Special Populations Tests

McNeil claims although sucralose is derived from sucrose, the body does not recognize it as a carbohydrate, as it would for native sucrose. "Sucralose does not effect normal carbohydrate metabolism, including insulin secretion and glucose and fructose absorption," they state. Sucralose is therefore suitable for consumption by the diabetic population.

Short-term glucose homeostatic effects of a single 1,000 mg sucralose (versus cellulose placebo) oral dose upon 13 insulin dependent diabetes mellitus (IDDM) and 13 non-insulin dependent diabetes mellitus (NIDDM) human subjects were observed.[28] All subjects had initial blood glucose levels within normal ranges. The average sucralose dose was 13.8 mg/kg for IDDM subjects and 10.5 mg/kg for NIDDM subject. All doses were in excess of the estimated daily sucralose intake at the 90th percentile (2.3 mg/kg). Results indicated that sucralose had no short-term adverse effects on blood glucose control in both IDDM and NIDDM diabetics. Similarly, sucralose contains no phenylalanine or other amino acids. Unlike aspartame, sucralose poses no risk to phenylketonuria patients.

#5: Corporate Animal And Clinical Studies From Tate & Lyle's Corporate Study[29]: Repeated dose study of sucralose tolerance in human subjects

Note: These studies were performed and submitted for review by Tate & Lyle (the creators of sucralose). This study was over a three-month period, and <u>fasting was indicated</u>, unlike the studies submitted to the FDA by McNeil.

Abbreviations: ADI=acceptable daily intake; EDI=estimated daily intake; HNEL=highest-no-effect level.

Abstract:

Two tolerance studies were conducted in healthy human adult volunteers. The first study was an ascending dose study conducted in eight subjects, in which sucralose was administered at doses of 1, 2.5, 5 and 10 mg/kg at forty-eight-hour intervals and followed by daily dosing at 2 mg/kg for three days and 5 mg/kg for 4 days. In the second study, subjects consumed either sucralose (n=77) or fructose (50 g/day) (n=31) twice daily in single blind fashion. Sucralose dosage levels were 125 mg/day for weeks 1–3, 250 mg/day during weeks 4–7, and 500 mg/day during weeks 8–12. No adverse experiences or clinically detectable effects were attributable to sucralose in either study.

Similarly, haematology, serum biochemistry, urinalysis and EKG tracings were unaffected by sucralose administration. In the 13-week study, serial slit lamp ophthalmologic examination performed in a random subset of the study groups revealed no changes. Fasting and 2-hour post-dosing blood sucralose concentrations obtained daily during week 12 of the study revealed no rising trend for blood sucralose. Sucralose was well tolerated by human volunteers in single doses up to 10 mg/kg/day and repeated doses increasing to 5 mg/kg/day for 13 weeks. <u>Based on these studies and the extensive animal safety database, there is no indication that adverse effects on human health would occur from frequent or long-term exposure to sucralose at the maximum anticipated levels of intake</u>.

#6: Toxins In Sucralose: A Brief Explanation of Toxins in Sucralose – Sulfuryl Chloride and Lithium Chloride

Note: As I wrote in Chapter One, according to the Splenda International Patent A23L001-236 and PEP Review #90-1-4 (July 1991), sucralose is synthesized by this five-step process:

1. Sucrose is tritylated with **trityl chloride** in the presence of **dimethylformamide** and **4-methylmorpholine** and the tritylated sucrose is then acetylated with **acetic anhydride**,
2. The resulting TRISPA (6,1',6'-tri-O-trityl-penta-O-acetylsucrose) is chlorinated with **hydrogen chloride** in the presence of **toluene**,
3. The resulting 4-PAS (sucrose 2,3,4,3',4'-pentaacetate) is heated in the presence of **methyl isobutyl ketone** and **acetic acid**,
4. The resulting 6-PAS (sucrose 2,3,6,3',4'-pentaacetate) is chlorinated with **thionyl chloride** in the presence of **toluene** and **benzyltriethylammonium chloride**, and
5. The resulting TOSPA (sucralose pentaacetate) is treated

with **methanol** (wood alcohol, a poison) in the presence of **sodium methoxide** to produce sucralose.

According to the abstract in the international patent for sucralose, 2,3,4,6, 3',4',6'-Hepta-O-acetylsucrose was treated with sulfuryl chloride (SO2Cl2) and the 1'-chlorosulfate was treated with lithium chloride (LiCl).[30] The following information is on sulfuryl chloride and lithium:

A. Sulfuryl Chloride (SO2Cl2)

Identifications:

- Formula: SO2Cl2
- Elements: Chlorine, Oxygen, Sulfur
- CAS Chemical Number: 7791-25-5
- Synonyms:
    - Chlorosulfuric acid
    - Sulfonyl chloride
    - Sulfonyl dichloride
    - Sulfonyl dichloride (SO2Cl2)
    - Sulfuric dichloride
    - Sulfuric oxychloride
    - Sulfuryl Chloride
    - Sulfuryl chloride (SO2Cl2)
    - Sulfuryl dichloride
    - Sulphuryl chloride

Health & Regulatory Guidelines

- NFPA 704 Rating:
    - Health Hazardard Rating: 3
    - Fire Hazardard Rating: 0
    - Reactivity Hazardard Rating: 2
- Corrosive: Yes
- Risk of Skin Injury: Yes [31]

B. Lithium From Lithium Chloride

- Discoverer: Johann Arfvedson
- Discovery Location: Sweden
- Discovery Year: 1817
- Name Origin: Greek: lithos (stone)
- Sources: spodumene, ambylgonite, lepidolite and desert lake brines. Also obtained by passing electric charge through melted lithium chloride.
- Uses: Used in batteries, ceramics, glass, lubricants, alloy hardeners, pharmaceuticals, hydrogenating agents, heat transfer liquids, rocket propellants, vitamin A synthesis, nuclear reactor coolant, underwater buoyancy devices and the production of tritium. Deoxidizer in copper and copper alloys.
- Additional Notes: Near its melting point, lithium ignites in air. Lithium posses a dangerous fire and explosion risk when exposed to water, acids or oxidizing agents. It reacts exothermally with nitrogen in moist air at high temperatures. In solution lithium is toxic and targets the central nervous system.

In both situations, the products ($ClCH2X$) arise by rapid nucleophilic displacement of the chlorosulfate molecule; this, then, more slowly liberates the chloride ion to enhance the production of sucralose.[32]

#7: Splenda Study Submitted To Canadian Government - Trichlorogalactosucrose – Sucralose[33]

The first draft of this condensed research report was prepared by Dr. D.L. Grant, Toxicological Evaluation Division Health and Welfare Canada. Sucralose had been evaluated previously by the 33rd Joint FAO/WHO Expert Committee on Food Additives in 1989. The Committee allocated a temporary ADI of 0-3.5 mg/kg bw, and indicated that further studies or information were required. For the entire research report, visit the following link: http://europa.eu.int/comm/food/fs/sc/scf/out68_en.pdf (See Appendix VIII.)

These research submissions spawned further concern by the American FDA when McNeil Specialties applied for FDA approval of Splenda, which are addressed within this chapter.

As I wrote in Chapter One, Splenda's chemical formal reads: 1,6-dichloro-1, 6-dideoxy-BETA-D-fructofuranosyl-4-chloro-4-deoxy-alpha-D-galactopyranoside. (Also, see Appendix I) This research report documents the results of a short-term rat study on Trichlorogalactose (TGS) also known as sucralose (1,6-dichloro-1,6-dideoxy-beta-D-fructo-furanosyl-4-chloro-4-deoxy-alpha-D-galactopyranoside) derived from sucrose by selective replacement of three hydroxy groups by chlorine atoms at positions 4', 1' and 6', which greatly increases sweetness. The research results are underlined throughout the report.

1. Explanation

Trichlorogalactosucrose (TGS) has been evaluated previously by the 33rd Joint FAO/WHO Expert Committee on Food Additives in 1989. [30] The Committee allocated a temporary ADI of 0-3.5 mg/kg bw, and indicated that the following further studies or information were required:

1. Information on the absorption and metabolism of TGS in humans after prolonged oral dosing.
2. Results of studies to ensure that TGS produces no adverse effects in people with insulin-dependent and maturity-onset diabetes.
3. Results of further studies in rats on the elimination of TGS from pregnant animals and from the fetus, to exclude the possibility of bioaccumulation.

Results of a short-term rat study on 6-chlorofructose. Trichlorogalactose (1,6-dichloro-1,6-dideoxy-beta-D-fructo-furanosyl-4-chloro-4-deoxy-alpha-D-galactopyranoside)(TG S),is derived from sucrose by selective replacement of the three hydroxy groups at positions 4',1' and 6' by chlorine atoms, which greatly increases sweetness.

At room temperature, in water, TGS is 600-650 times sweeter than sucrose at a concentration of 4-5%. In acid solution, TGS hydrolyses slowly to its constituent monosaccharides, 4-chlorogalactose (4-CG) and 1,6-dichlorofructose(1,6-DCF). This process is influenced by temperature and pH. Under the extreme conditions (treatment of TGS with 0.11N aqueous hydrochloric acid at 68 °C for 72 h) used to produce sufficient quantities of 4CG and 1,6-DCF for toxicological testing, an aqueous solution was obtained composed of: 1,6-dichlorofructose (47.5%); 4-chlorogalactose (49.1%); 6-chlorofructose (0.3%); 1-chlorofructose (0.2%) and TGS (1.2%).

Since the previous evaluation, the results of additional studies and additional information have become available. At the present meeting, the Committee evaluated new and existing data that are summarized and discussed in the following addendum to the monograph.

2. Biological Data

2.1 Special study on palatability

2.1.1 Rat Groups of 10 female Sprague-Dawley, CD strain rats had free access to two bottles containing either tap water or TGS solution at concentrations ranging from 20 2560 mg/ml for 32 days. Rats showed a range of individual variability in their preference for TGS vs. water. As a group, however, they displayed a distinct preference for TGS over water at concentrations up to 320 mg/100 ml. At concentrations above 640 mg/100 ml, water was preferred over the TGS solution. There was no mortality and no signs of clinical toxicity were observed (Amyes & Aughton, 1987).

Groups of 20 young female Sprague-Dawley rats, Crl: CDBR strain had access to two feeding jars containing either basal diet or a mixture of basal diet containing TGS. The starting concentration of TGS was 50 ppm and was doubled every fourth day to a final concentration of 3200 ppm (32 days). No statistically significant difference in the selection of basal diet or TGS containing diet was observed at 50 or 100 ppm. A statistically significant preference for TGS diet was observed at 200 ppm. At the 400 ppm concentration, basal and TGS-containing diets were consumed in similar amounts. At TGS concentration of 800 ppm or higher, a

statistically significant preference was displayed for basal diet. The total intake of food by treated rats was similar to that of their controls. No death, nor apparent effect on the appearance, behavior, or body weight was reported (Amyes & Aughton, 1988).

2.2 Short-term studies

2.2.1 Rat Groups of Sprague-Dawley rats were given TGS (dissolved in water) by gavage at dose levels of 4000 mg/kg bw/day (15 rats/sex)for periods of 4, 9, or 13 weeks, respectively. Corresponding control groups (receiving water) with the same number of animals as the treated groups were included. <u>A significant increase of caecal weights was observed in rats of both sexes at all dose levels. Sporadic significant changes in some parameters of haematology and clinical chemistry and some differences in organ weights (in some groups at some time points) were observed.</u> The changes were not clearly dose-related and not considered as treatment-related. Other investigated parameters were not adversely affected, these included: clinical signs of toxicity, mortality, body weight gains, food and water consumption, urinalysis, gross and histopathology (Perry *et al.,*1988). 4-CHLOROGALACTOSE(4-CG) and 1,6-DICHLOROFRUCTOSE (1,6-DCF)

Biological Data

No information available.

2.2 Toxicological studies

2.2.1 Special studies on neurotoxicity

2.2.2.1 Mouse
Groups of male CD-1 mice (8 mice/group) were dosed daily (by gavage) with 6-chlorofructose (6-CF) (one of the TGS hydrolysis products obtained by treating TGS with aqueous hydrochloric acid [0.11N] at 68°C for 72 h) at dose levels of 240 or 480 mg/kg b.w. day for 28 days. Mice were weighed daily and examined for hind limb paralysis at the same time. Negative control group animals were given water while positive controls received 6-chloroglucose (6-CG) at a level of 480 mg/kg bw/day. The results showed that 6-CF at both dose levels **caused dose-related hind-limb paralysis in some treated animals** (240 mg/kg bw/day: 2/8; 480 mg/kg bw/day: 7/8) starting between 4 to 6 days post-dosing (Ford & Waites, 1982).

2.2.3 Special studies on reproduction

2.2.3.1 Rat Groups of mature male CD rats (3-8 rats/group) were exposed orally to 6-CF at dose levels of 6, 12, 18, or 48 mg/kg bw/day for 14 days. Treated male rats were mated with untreated females during the final 7 days of dosing. Mated females were killed 10 days after mating and live embryos, resorptions and the corpora lutea were counted. The results showed that males exposed to 6-CF at dose levels of 18 or 48 mg/kg bw/day became infertile (conception rate: control - 79%;

treated groups - 0%). <u>Three weeks after cessation of treatment the conception rates had recovered to the level of control groups.</u> The lowest dose level of 6 mg/kg/b.w./day did not have any adverse effect on the fertility of male rats (Ford & Waites, 1978a; Ford *et al.,* 1981; Ford & Waites, 1982).

Three groups of male Sprague Dawley rats of the CD strain (6 rats/group) were given 6-chlorofructose dissolved in water by gavage twice daily at dose levels of 0, 3 or 9 mg/kg b.w./day for 10 weeks. An additional group consisting of 6 males received 6-chlorofructose twice daily at a level of 27 mg/kg bw/day for 4 weeks. After 7 days of treatment, males were paired on a one-to-one basis with untreated females. Each morning the females were examined for copulation plugs and presence of spermatozoa in a vaginal smear. Quantity and quality of spermatozoa were assessed. Females that had not conceived during the first four days of pairing were sacrificed and their reproductive organs examined. The pairing procedure was repeated at weekly intervals for 10 or for 8 weeks except for males of the 27 mg/kg bw/day dose group which were paired weekly for 4 weeks. Males were observed daily for signs of clinical toxicity and mating behavior. Body weight gains were recorded weekly. After completing the series of matings, the males were killed, necropsied, and the following organs weighed: testes, epididymis, prostate and seminal vesicle. Testes and epididymis of the control and 9 mg/kg bw/day dose groups were histopathologically examined. On days 8-10 *post coitum,* females were sacrificed and the uterine horns checked for the presence of implantation sites. For each male, mating performance, conception rate and fertility index were calculated.

<u>**Males** receiving 27 mg/kg b.w./day became **infertile for the entire treatment period** (4 weeks), but regained their fertility within the first 7 days of recovery period. Females mated by males of the 9 mg/kg bw/day dose group showed a reduction in the number of implantation sites, **indicating a possible decrease**</u>

in male fertility. The fertility of males of the 3 mg/kg bw/day dose group was not affected (Tesh,*et al.,* 1984).

Acute toxicity TGS-HP

Species	Sex	Route	LD50 (mg/kg bw)	Reference
Rat	female	oral	4450	Campbell et al. 1980

Comments

At its present meeting, the Committee reviewed new and previously available data. Although no new data on the absorption and metabolism of TGS in humans were received, the Committee concluded that there was no indication that these processes would change on prolonged oral dosing. This conclusion was drawn from the comparative metabolic data for TGS in various species, including humans, and the lack of evidence of toxicity in extensive animal studies. **Nevertheless, the Committee recognized that the data did not address all possibilities, particularly the potential effects of adaptation of the gastrointestinal microflora.**

No specific studies on possible adverse effects of TGS in people with insulin-dependent and maturity-onset diabetes had been performed. However, the Committee decided that this concern could be satisfactorily addressed through consideration of data that showed that TGS had no effect on the secretion of insulin in humans or rats, blood glucose levels or carbohydrate metabolism. Furthermore, the Committee was aware of proposed studies involving both types of diabetics.

On re-assessment of the overall data on TGS, including

the metabolic data in various species, including humans and pregnant and non-pregnant rabbits, and in the absence of any significant finding in the two-generation reproduction study in rats, the Committee concluded that the question on the accumulation of TGS in pregnant animals and fetuses was satisfactorily addressed, and that there was no evidence to suggest a difference in metabolism in pregnant and non-pregnant animals.

The Committee reviewed additional studies relating to the possible toxicity of the potential breakdown product of TGS,6-chlorofructose (in sucralose). In a short-term study (28 days) in which 6-chlorofructose was administered at 240 and 480 mg per kg of body weight per day, **male mice showed hind-limb paralysis**. In addition, three special studies were conducted to assess reproductive function in rats. **Administration of 6-chlorofructose at 18-48 mg per kg of body weight per day for 7-14 days caused a loss of fertility in male rats**. In two of these studies, the no-effect-levels were 3 and 6 mg per kg of body weight (bw) per day. The Committee noted, however, that 6-chlorofructose is only a potential breakdown product of TGS.

40 or 480 mg/kg bw day for 28 days. Mice were weighed daily and examined for hind limb paralysis at the same time. Negative control group animals were given water while positive controls received 6-chloroglucose (6-CG) at a level of 480 mg/kg bw/day. The results showed that 6-CF at both dose levels caused dose-related hind-limb paralysis in some treated animals (240 mg/kg bw/day: 2/8; 480 mg/kg bw/day: 7/8) starting between 4 to 6 days post-dosing (Ford & Waites, 1982).

CHAPTER 9

Sneak Peeks Into Little-Known Sweetener Facts

- In 1850, Americans consumed about thirteen ounces of soda per person a year. In the late 1980s, more than 500 twelve-ounce cans of sodas were consumed per person each year. The 1994 annual report of the beverage industry showed that per-capita consumption of sodas was 49.1 gallons per year. Of this amount, 28.2 percent of consumption was diet soda.

- A survey at the campus of Pennsylvania State University has shown that some students drank as much as fourteen cans of soda a day. One girl had consumed thirty-seven cokes in two days. Many admitted they could not live without soft drinks. If deprived, they developed withdrawal symptoms much like those addicted to drugs.

- For the four weeks ending January 26, 2004, Splenda's dollar-market share of the tabletop-sweetener market exceeded that of Equal-brand products for the first time, 29.7 percent to 27.2 percent, according to Information Resources Inc., a Chicago-based concern that tracks CPG sales in all mass-market stores except Wal-Mart. Sweet N' Low sugar substitutes remained in third place, with a 19.5 percent market share. Those numbers further displayed momentum that began last year, when Splenda's dollar sales rose about 69 percent while Equal's fell by 8 percent and Sweet'N Low's rose 1 percent.

- In 2000, Monsanto sold its sweetener business that included NutraSweet, for $440 million.

- Carbonated soft drinks account for more than 27 percent of America's beverage consumption.

- By 1997, Americans spent over $54 billion to buy fourteen billion gallons of soft drinks. That is equivalent to more than 576 12-ounce servings per year or 1.6 12-ounce cans per day for every man, woman, and child - more than twice the amount produced in 1974.

- Artificially-sweetened diet sodas accounted for twenty-four percent of cola sales, up from 8.6% in 1970.

- One fifth of one- and two-year-old children consume soft drinks daily, drinking an average of seven ounces -- nearly one cup -- per day.

- Approximately one-half of all children between six and eleven drink soft drinks.

- One-fourth of thirteen- to eighteen-year-old male cola drinkers consumes 2 1/2 or more cans per day. One out of twenty drinks five cans or more a day. One-fourth of thirteen- to eighteen-year-old female cola drinkers consumes about two or more cans per day, and one out of twenty drinks three cans or more a day. By contrast, twenty years ago, the typical thirteen- to eighteen- year-old consumer of soft drinks (boys and girls together) drank 3/4 of a can per day.

- May 2004, Coca-Cola started building its first factory in China's northwestern region, and its 25th bottling plant in China, with an investment of twelve million US dollars. With an annual capacity of twenty-four million cases, the new plant was put into operation in Lanzhou, capital of Gansu Province, by the end of 2004.

- Harvey Weinstein, CEO of the Miramax empire, rides in a limo stocked with Diet Coke. John Edwards, failed presidential candidate, has been known to drink as many as ten Diet Cokes while campaigning -- a habit endorsed wholeheartedly by both of the Clintons.

- The FAA discourages pilots from drinking diet drinks while they are in flight because aspartame has been known to cause blackouts and seizures during changes in air pressure.

- Splenda representatives have put forth two primary arguments to defend the claim that sucralose is not toxic nor causes health problems in laboratory experiments:
  1. The dose of sucralose in laboratory experiments was high.
  2. The sucralose was unpleasant for the rodents to eat in large doses. They claim that starvation caused the shruken thymus glands.

- FDA Rules and Regulations Federal Register Report Vol. 63, No. 64, 16426 shows a problem with sucralose causing caecal enlargement and renal mineralization, shrunken thymus glands, and other questionable health reactions to sucralose seen in post mortem animal research.

- Seven laboratory animal deaths occurred during the studies submitted to the FDA by McNeil Nutritionals, attributed either to spontaneous causes not related to treatment, or to technical trauma during dosing,

- The seven animal deaths in the McNeil laboratory studies have been left "unresolved."

- In the McNeil studies, water consumption was significantly higher in the sucralose-treated rats as compared to the control rats.

- Sucralose is a simple sugar.

- Hydrolysis of sucralose can occur under conditions of prolonged storage at elevated temperatures in highly acidic aqueous food products. Therefore, sucralose can break down in heat (not specified at what temperature) in acidic solutions *such as a cola can*, and when stored for a prolonged time period.

- McNeil launched Splenda directly to consumers as a tabletop and cooking sweetener in 2000. Demand outstripped supply within a few months, so the company pulled back on marketing until after its new Splenda plant in Alabama opened in 2001. Since then, Splenda has launched a blistering marketing assault on Equal and Sweet N' Low.

- According to the numbers, Equal has taken a much bigger hit from Splenda in terms of market share than Sweet 'N Low because Sweet 'N Low is priced much lower than Splenda and Equal, yet appears to remain the number one-selling brand in terms of units and volume.

- Chicago-based Merisant Corp. is the latest manufacturer

of NutraSweet/ Equal.

- Chlorine at water treatment plants is unstable and easily separates from the water as free-form chlorine, which can be a carcinogen.

- POPs have one final fatal flaw — *an attachment to fat.* Human and animal fatty tissues absorb POPs. United Nations Environmental Program (UNEP) scientists state that in some animals, POPs have been detected at levels 70,000 times higher than in their surroundings.

- Studies have demonstrated exposure to chlorine increases the risk of cancer and birth defects among wildlife. They provoke allergic reactions and damage the nervous, reproductive and immune systems of animals.

- Some dioxins and organochlorines mimic the hormone estrogen, thus altering wildlife in ways that diminish their "ability and interest" in producing offspring.

- All samples of Pepsi® and Coca-Cola® tested in the CSE and public laboratories in India were found to have the presence of deadly pesticide residues. The pesticides, which were found in soft drink samples, were DDT, Lindane, Chlorphyrifos and Malathion; all pose long-term health hazards.

- Researchers above stated that the presence of the pesticides in the Indian samples was higher than the European Union (EU) standards. In Indian Coca Cola, the presence of pesticides was 45 times higher than EU standards, in Fanta® 43 times, in Mirinda Orange® 39 times, in Limca® 30 times, in Pepsi 30 times, in 7-Up® 33 times, in Blue Pepsi® 29 times, in Mountain Dew® 28 times, in Thumbs Up® 22 times, in Diet Coke® 14 times, and in Sprite® 11 times higher than EU standards.

- The Indian Tamilnadu Traders Union has urged the Congress-led government at the Centre to seriously reconsider the World Trade Agreement and implement a ban on multi-national soft drinks including Coke and Pepsi. The Prime Minister was urged to pass legislation banning multi-national soft drinks including Coke and Pepsi, which they state are scientifically proven to contain harmful pesticides.

- All soft drinks may soon be replaced with fruit juices and water in Regina, Canada public schools. Regina's public school board is debated what beverages should be allowed in school vending machines. Board policy currently allows the schools to sign exclusive contracts with soft drink companies, which provide additional revenue for the schools.

CHAPTER 10

The Sweetener Wars

There is a unseen battle going on in the sweetener industry for the consumer's dollar, and your understanding of these sweetener products can influence your health. Huge corporations are competing against one another for dominance in this market, so who *will* win this trendy, multi-billion dollar sweetener war?

Every day we consumers are bombarded with advertising's seductive messages: *this product will make you beautiful, thin, and happy - eat all you want with no complications – sugar-free is the solution to your child's behavior problems.* We constantly internalize these messages on TV, radio, billboards and magazines. Now many people have been convinced that chemical sugar-free sweeteners are actually healthy for them.

In this incredible age of high-speed information, we need to discern the source of our health information. Who do we listen to – big business or concerned natural health professionals? The current cultural trends of thinness and endless youth are fueling "pseudo-information."

Confused by who and what to believe? Consider this: artificial manmade chemicals can negatively impact your body just as most manmade chemicals damage the natural environment. Foods produced by nature actually feed your body, creating health.

So, who will win this sweetener war? Hopefully, with good information and a natural diet, <u>YOU</u> will win! It's your choice.

Appendix I
Splenda's Chemical Formula

Chemical Name

Alpha-D-Galactopyranoside,1,6-dichloro-1,6-dideoxy-beta-D-fructofuranosyl 4-chloro-4-deoxy-(9Cl) (CA INDEX NAME)

1',4',6'-Trichloro-galacto-sucrose
4,1',6'-Trichloro-4,1'6'-trideoxygalactosucrose

The chemical tag for sucralose is 1,6-dichloro-1, 6-dideoxy-BETA-D-fructofuranosyl-4-chloro-4-deoxy-alpha-<u>D-galactopyranoside</u>. But traditionally, a product made from sugar should have the chemical tag 1,6-dichloro-1, 6-dideoxy-BETA-D-fructofuranosyl-4-chloro-4-deoxy-alpha-D-<u>glucopyranoside</u>. As it appears, sucralose is a <u>D-galactopyranoside</u> and not a <u>D-glucopyranoside</u> if considered to be real sugar.

Abstract

Chlorinated sucroses 1(R=Cl, R1=OH, R2=H, R3, R4=OH, Cl; R=R1=R3=R4=Cl, R2=H) and galactosucroses 1(R=OH, Cl, R1=H, R2=Cl, R3, R4=OH, Cl) have a sweetening power 4-2000 times that of sucrose.

2,3,4,6,3',4',6' – Hepta-O-acetylsucrose was treated with SO2Cl2 and the 1'-chlorosulfate treated with LiCl and deblocked to give 1(R=Cl, R1=R3=R4=OH, R2=H

Appendix II
FDA Final Rule Report Sucralose (Splenda)

Federal Register: August 12, 1999 (Volume 64, Number 155)
Rules and Regulations
Page 43908-43909

From the Federal Register Online via GPO Access [wais.access.gpo.gov]
DOCID: fr12au99-5

Department Of Health And Human Service

Food and Drug Administration
21 CFR Part 172
Docket No. 99F-0001

Food Additives Permitted for Direct Addition to Food for Human

Consumption; Sucralose

AGENCY: Food and Drug Administration, HHS.

ACTION: Final rule.

SUMMARY: The Food and Drug Administration (FDA) is amending the food additive regulations to provide for the safe use of sucralose as a general purpose sweetener for food. This action is in response to a petition filed by McNeil Specialty Products Co.

DATES: This regulation is effective August 12, 1999; written objections and requests for a hearing by September 13, 1999.

ADDRESSES: Written objections may be sent to the Dockets Management
Branch (HFA-305), Food and Drug Administration, 5630 Fishers Lane, rm.
1061, Rockville, MD 20852.

FOR FURTHER INFORMATION CONTACT: Blondell Anderson, Center for Food Safety and Applied Nutrition (HFS-206), Food and Drug Administration, 200 C St. SW., Washington, DC 20204, 202-418-3106.

Supplementary Information:

I. Introduction

In a notice published in the Federal Register on January 11, 1999 (64 FR 1634), FDA announced that a food additive petition (FAP 8A4624) had been filed by McNeil Specialty Products, Co., 501 George St., New Brunswick, NJ 08903-2400. The petition proposed that the food additive regulations be amended at Sec. 172.831 (21 CFR 172.831) to expand the permitted uses of sucralose to allow for use as a general purpose sweetener in food. FDA previously approved sucralose for use in 15 food categories under Sec. 172.831 (64 FR 16417, April 3, 1998).

II. Identity

Sucralose is a disaccharide that is made from sucrose in a five-step process that selectively substitutes three atoms of chlorine for three hydroxyl groups in the sugar molecule. It is a free-flowing, white crystalline solid, product at an approximate purity of 98 percent, that is soluble in water and stable both in crystalline form and in most aqueous solutions. The sweetness intensity for sucralose in 320 to 1,000 times that of sucrose, depending on the food application.

Hydrolysis of sucralose may occur under conditions of prolonged storage at elevated temperatures in highly acidic aqueous food products. The hydrolysis products are the monosaccharides, 4-chloro-4-deoxy-galactose (4-CG) and 1,6-dichloro-1,6-dideoxyfructose (1,6-DCF).

III. Evaluation of Safety

In support of safety for the proposed expanded uses of sucralose, the petitioner referenced the toxicological safety data base submitted in food additive petition (FAP) 9A3987 that established the safety of the currently approved uses. Also referenced were the identity, manufacturing process, and specifications for the sweetener. In the new petition (FAP 8A4624), the petitioner submitted data concerning:
Use and typical use levels;

1. self-limiting levels; (3) proof of technical effect
2. exposure
3. stability
4. analysis in foods for both sucralose and its potential hydrolysis products

In order to determine whether sucralose can be safety used as a general [[Page 43909]] purpose sweetener, the agency reevaluated the currently established acceptable daily intake (ADI) for sucralose, 5 milligrams per kilogram body weight per day (mg/kg bw/d) (Ref. 1) and determined that this ADI is still appropriate (Ref. 2). FDA also estimated new daily intakes (EDI) for the 90th percentile consumer of sucralose to include the expanded uses. The new EDI was derived from projections based on the amount of sucralose that may be used in the currently regulated food categories, the proposed food categories, and on data regarding the consumption levels of these particular foods. Based upon the data in the petition and other information, the agency established a no effect level (NOEL) for the hydrolysis products of sucralose at 30 mg/kg bw/d (Ref. 2).

To aid in the establishment of new exposure estimates for sucralose and its hydrolysis products, the petitioner submitted a Market Research Corporation of America (MRCA) report that addresses foods in which sucralose may be used and an updated report on the potential exposure for the hydrolysis products. From this information, the agency has determined that based on the expanded uses, the cumulative exposure to sucralose could increase to 2.4 mg/kg bw/d and the cumulative exposure to its hydrolysis products to 0.007 mg/kg bw/d (Ref. 3). The agency concludes: Exposure to sucralose will remain below the previously established ADI of 5.0 mg/kg bw/d for sucralose, and exposure to the hydrolysis products will remain far below the no effect level of 30 mg/kg bw/d (Refs. 2 and 3).

IV. Conclusions
From the review of all the information available on sucralose and its hydrolysis products, the agency concludes that sucralose may be safely used as a sweetener in food generally (Refs. 2 and 3).

In accordance with Sec. 171.1(h) (21 CFR 171.1(h)), the petition and the documents that FDA considered and relied upon in reaching its decision to approve the petition are available for inspection at the Center for Food Safety and Applied Nutrition by appointment with the information contact person listed above. As provided in Sec. 171.1(h), the agency will delete from the documents any materials that are not available for public disclosure before making the documents available for inspection.

V. Environmental
The agency has carefully considered the potential environmental effects of this action. FDA has concluded that

the action will not have a significant impact on the human environment, and that an environmental impact statement is not required. The agency's finding of no significant impact and the evidence supporting that finding, contained in an environmental assessment, may be seen in the Dockets Management Branch (address above) between 9 a.m. and 4 p.m., Monday through Friday.

VI. Paperwork Reduction Act 1995

This final rule contains no collection of information. Therefore, clearance by the Office of Management and Budget under the Paperwork Reduction Act of 1995 is not required.

VII. Objections

Any person who will be adversely affected by this regulation may at any time on or before September 13, 1999, file with the Dockets Management Branch (address above) written objections thereto. Each objection shall be separately numbered, and each numbered objection shall specify with particularly the provisions of the regulation to which objection is made and the grounds for the objection. Each numbered objection on which a hearing is requested shall specifically so state. Failure to request a hearing for any particular objection shall constitute a waiver of the right to a hearing on that objection.

Each numbered objection for which a hearing is requested shall include a detailed description and analysis of the specific factual information intended to be presented in support of the objection in the event that hearing is held. Failure to include such a description and analysis for any particular objection shall constitute a waiver of the right to a hearing on the objection. Three copies of all documents shall be submitted and shall be identified with the docket number found in brackets in the heading of this document. Any objections received in response to the regulation may be seen in the Dockets Management Branch between 9 a.m. and 4 p.m., Monday through Friday.

VIII. References

The following references have been placed on display in the Dockets Management Branch (address above) and may be seen by interested persons between 9 a.m. and 4 p.m., Monday through Friday.

1. Addendum memorandum from Whiteside, Scientific Support Branch,FDA, to Anderson, Novel Ingredients Branch, FDA, November 13, 1997.

2. Memorandum from Whiteside, Division of Health Effects Evaluation, FDA, to Anderson, Regulatory Policy Branch, February 25, 1999.

3. Memorandum from DiNovi, Division Product Manufacture and Use, FDA, to Anderson, Division of Product Policy, FDA, October 22, 1998.

List of Subjects in 21 CFR Part 172 Food additives, Reporting and recordkeeping requirements. Therefore, under the Federal Food, Drug, and Cosmetic Act and under authority delegated to the Commissioner of Food and Drugs, 21 CFR part 172 is amended as follows:

Part 172 - Food Additives Permitted For Direct Addition To Food For Human Consumption

1. The authority citation for 21 CFR part 172 continues to read as follows:

Authority: 21 U.S.C. 321, 341, 342, 348, 371, 379e.

2. Section 172.831 is amended by removing the introductory paragraph and by revising paragraph (c) to read as follows: Sec. 172.831 Sucralose.

Appendix II – FDA Final Rule Report Sucralose (Splenda)

* * * * *

(a) ***
(b) ***
(c) The additive may be used as a sweetener in foods generally, in accordance with current good manufacturing practice in an amount not to exceed that reasonably required to accomplish the intended effect.

* * * * *

Dated: August 5, 1999. Margaret M. Dotzel, Acting Associate Commissioner for Policy. [FR Doc. 99-20888 Filed 8-11-99; 8:45 am] BILLING CODE 4160-01-F

Appendix III
Splenda Patent Registrations

1. Patent Stereochemistry

Sucralose (Trichloro-galacto-sucrose / chlorinated sucrose) was approved by the American FDA in 1988 as a tabletop sweetener and for use in a number of desserts, confections, and nonalcoholic beverages.

The following information is recorded directly from Splenda's patent registration, CAS Registry Number 56038-13-2:

Chemical Name
Alpha-D-Galactopyranoside,1,6-dichloro-1,6-dideoxy-beta-D-fructofuranosyl 4-chloro-4-deoxy-(9Cl) (CA INDEX NAME)

1',4',6'-Trichloro-galacto-sucrose
4,1',6'-Trichloro-4,1'6'-trideoxygalactosucrose

Splenda
Sucralose

Molecular Formula
$C12H19Cl3O8$

2. International Patent

A second patent report is filed in the CAS Registry: International Patent Classification A23L001-236

Title
Chlorinated sucrose sweeteners

Inventor Name
Leslie Hough, Shashikant Purushottam Phadnis, Riaz Ahmed, Michael Ralph Jenner

Patent Assignee
Tate & Lyle Ltd, England

Publication Source
Ger. Offen, 27 pp

Patent Names And Dates
Priority Application Information

Country	Patent #	Date
GB	1976-616	January 8, 1976
GB	1976-19570	May 12, 1976
CA	1976-268863	December 29, 1976
US	1976-755661	December 30, 1976
AT	1977-48	January 7, 1977

Abstract
Chlorinated sucroses 1(R=Cl, R1=OH, R2=H, R3, R4=OH, Cl; R=R1=R3=R4=Cl, R2=H) and galactosucroses 1(R=OH, Cl, R1=H, R2=Cl, R3, R4=OH, Cl) have a sweetening power 4-2000 times that of sucrose.

2,3,4,6,3',4',6' – Hepta-O-acetylsucrose was treated with

SO2Cl2 and the 1'-chlorosulfate treated with LiCl and deblocked to give 1(R=Cl, R1=R3=R4=OH, R2=H

3. A Third Report Filed in the CAS Registry

Title
 History and development of sucralose by Samuel V. Molinary and Mike R. Jenner 182, 6-15

 Tate & Lyle Specialty Sweeteners, White Knights, Reading, RG6 60X, UK

Public Source
 Food Ingredients J. Jpn. (1999)

Abstract
Molinary and Jenner write (sic): A review with fifteen references was submitted. Sucralose was discovered during a collaborative research program between Tate & Lyle and Queen Elizabeth College of the University of London. It is made by selective substitution of sucralose hydroxyl groups by chlorine, resulting in a highly intense (600 times) sugar-like sweetness and in exceptional chemical stability at both high temperatures and low pH. This report describes the research leading to the discovery and subsequent development of sucralose, and the manufacturing processes are discussed in addition to its regulatory status worldwide.

Appendix IV
International Life Sciences Institute (ILSI) Members

Complete ILSI Member List [Sweetener Companies in bold (sic)]

Members Of ILSI

ILSI Argentina

Adams S.A.
Coca-Cola de Argentina S.A.
Danone S.A.
Kellogg's Argentina, S.A.
Kraft Foods Argentina
Kromberg
Merisant Argentina S.R.L.
Monsanto Argentina S.A.I.C.
PepsiCo de Argentina S.R.L.
Procter & Gamble Interaméricas Inc.
Refinería Hileret S.A.I.C.

ILSI Brasil

Abbott Laboratórios do Brasil
ADM do Brasil
Agripec Quimica e Farmaceutica S/A
Ajinomoto Interamericana Indústria e
Comércio Ltda.
BASF S.A.
Bayer CropScience Ltda.
Bristol-Myers Squibb Brasil S/A

Cadbury Adams Brasil Ind. e. Com. de
Produtos Alimentos Ltda.
Colloides Naturels Brasil
Comercial Ltda.
Danisco Brasil Ltda.
Danone Ltda.
Dow Agrosciences Industrial Ltda.
DSM Nutritional Products
FMC Química do Brasil
Herbalife International do Brasil Ltda.
Kraft Foods Brasil Ltda.
Masterfoods Brasil Alimentos Ltda.
Milenia Agro Ciências S.A.
Monsanto do Brasil Ltda.
Nestlé Brasil Ltda.
NutraSweet do Brasil Ltda.
Nutrimental S/A Indústria e Comércio de
Alimentos
ORAFTI LatinoAmerica Coordenação
Regional Ltda.
PepsiCo do Brasil Ltda.
Recofarma Indústria do Amazonas Ltda.
(Coca-Cola)
Red Bull do Brasil Ltda.
Sadia Concórdia S.A. Indústria e
Comércio
Sanavita Indústria e Comércio de
Alimentos Funcionais
Sensient Colors Brasil Ltda.
Solae do Brasil Ind. e Com. de
Alimentos Ltda.
Syngenta Proteçao de Cultivos Ltda.
Unilever Bestfoods Brasil
Yakult S.A. Indústria e Comércio

ILSI Europe

Acatris Holding
Ajinomoto Europe
Allied Domecq
Arla Foods
Barilla Alimentare
BASF
Bayer CropScience
Beverages Partners Worldwide
Brasseries Kronenbourg
Campina
Cereal Partners Worldwide
Cerestar
Coca-Cola Greater Europe
Cognis
Collöides Naturels International
Danisco Sweeteners
Diageo
Döhler Group
Dow Europe
DSM Food Specialties
DSM Nutritional Products
Ferrero Group
Firmenich
Friesland Coberco Dairy Foods
Frito-Lay Europe
GlaxoSmithKline
Groupe Danone
Heineken
Kellogg Company
Kraft Foods International
Masterfoods
McDonald's Corporation Quality
Assurance Europe
McNeil Consumer Nutritionals Europe

Monsanto Europe
Nestlé
NovoZymes
Nutrinova
Orkla Foods
Parmalat Italia
Procter & Gamble
Puleva Biotech
Raffinerie Tirlemontoise—ORAFTI
Raisio Group
Red Bull
RHM Technology
Roquette Frères
Royal Numico
Seven Seas
Südzucker
Swiss Quality Testing Services
Tate & Lyle Speciality Sweeteners
Tropicana Europe
Unilever
Valio
The Valspar Corporation
VK Mühlen
WILD Flavors/Ingredients
Yakult

ILSI Focal Point In China

(supporting companies)

Ajinomoto Co., Inc.
Akzo Nobel (Singapore)
Almond Board of California
Coca Cola (China) Beverage Co., Ltd.
Danisco (China) Co., Ltd. Beijing
Representative Office

Groupe Danone
Heinz-UFE Ltd.
International Flavours & Fragrances
(China) Ltd.
Kraft Foods, Beijing Nabisco Food
Co., Ltd.
Mars Incorporated
Monsanto Company
Nestlé (China) Ltd.
The NutraSweet Company
Nutrexpa - Cola Cao Tianjin Food
Co., Ltd.
Ocean Spray Cranberries, Inc.
Pepsico Inc. PepsiCo Hong Kong
The Procter & Gamble Company
Roche (China) Ltd.
Shanghai PepsiCo Snack Co., Ltd.
Frito-Lay China
Tate & Lyle Specialty Sweeteners
Unilever Bestfoods (China) Co., Ltd.
Wyeth-Ayerst (China) Limited

ILSI Health And Environmental Sciences Institute

3M Pharmaceuticals
Abbott Laboratories
Altana Pharma AG
Amgen, Inc.
AstraZeneca AB
ATOFINA Chemicals, Inc.
Aventis Pharmaceuticals
BASF Corporation
Bayer AG
Berlex Laboratories, Inc.

Biogen Idec MA Inc.
Boehringer Ingelheim GmbH
Bristol-Myers Squibb Company
Dow AgroSciences/The Dow Chemical
Company
E.I. du Pont de Nemours and Company
Eastman Kodak Company
Eisai Co., Ltd.
Eli Lilly and Company
Endo Pharmaceuticals
ExxonMobil Biomedical Sciences
GlaxoSmithKline
Hoffmann-La Roche, Inc.
Institute de Recherches Int. Servier
Johnson & Johnson Pharmaceuticals
L'Oreal Corporation
Meiji Seika Kaisha, Ltd.
Merck & Co., Inc.
Mitsubishi Pharma Corporation
Monsanto Company
N.V. Organon
Novartis Pharmaceuticals Corporation
Novo Nordisk A/S
Pfizer Inc.
The Procter & Gamble Company
Purdue Pharma L.P.
Rohm and Haas Company
Sankyo Co., Ltd.
Sanofi-Synthelabo Inc.
Schering-Plough Research Institute
Solvay Pharmaceuticals GmbH
Sumitomo Chemical Co., Ltd.
Syngenta
Tanabe Seiyaku Co., Ltd.
U.S. Borax, Inc.
Valent U.S.A. Corporation

Wyeth Research

ILSI India

Ajinomoto Co., Inc.
Akzo Nobel Chemicals Pte. Ltd.
Coca-Cola India
Ganesh Benzoplast Ltd.
General Mills India Pvt. Ltd.
Haldirams Marketing Pvt. Ltd.
Hindustan Lever Limited
ITC Foods Business
Kanmoor Foods Limited c/o Marico
Industries Limited
Kejriwal Enterprises
Mars Incorporated
Monsanto Enterprises Ltd.
National Dairy Development
Board
Nestlé India Limited
Nicholas Piramal India Limited
Roha Dyechem Ltd.
RSA Vitamins Private Limited
Sayaji Sethness Ltd.
The NutraSweet Company

ILSI Japan

Ajinomoto Co., Inc.
Ajinomoto General Foods, Inc.
AOHATA Corporation
API Co., Ltd.
ARSOA Honsha Corporation
Asahi Breweries Ltd.
Asahi Denka Kogyo K.K.
Coca-Cola (Japan) Co., Ltd.

Coca-Cola Asia Pacific Research & Development Co., Ltd.
Colloides Naturels Japan, Inc.
Danisco Japan Ltd.
DSM Nutrition Japan K.K.
Du Pont Kabushiki Kaisha
Ensuiko Sugar Refining Co., Ltd.
Fuji Oil Co., Ltd.
Guivaudan Japan K.K.
Hayashibara Biochemical
Laboratories, Inc.
Ikeda Tohka Industries Co., Ltd.
Inabata Koryo Co., Ltd.
International Flavors ü Fragrances
(Japan) Ltd.
Itoen, Ltd.
J.T. Food Business Division
Kaneka Corporation
KAO Corporation
Kellogg (Japan) K.K.
Kikkoman Corporation
Kirin Brewery Company, Limited
Knorr Foods Co., Ltd.
Kyowa Hakko Kogyo Co., Ltd.
Food Company
Lotte Co., Ltd.
Matsutani Chemical Industry
Co., Ltd.
Meiji Dairies Corporation
Meiji Seika Kaisha, Ltd.
Mitsubishi Materials Corporation
Mitsubishi-Kagaku Foods
Corporation
Mitsukan Co., Ltd.
Miyoshi Oil & Fat Co., Ltd.
Monsanto Japan Ltd.

Appendix IV – International Life Sciences Institute (ILSI) Members

Morinaga & Co., Ltd.
Morinaga Milk Industry Co., Ltd.
Nagaoka Perfumery Co., Ltd.
Nestlé Japan Manufacturing Ltd.
Nichirei Corporation
Nihon Shokuhin Kako Co., Ltd.
Nikken Foods Co., Ltd.
Nippon Flour Mills Co., Ltd.
Nippon Lever K.K.
Nippon Meat Packers, Inc.
Nisshin Oillio Group, Ltd.
Nisshin Seifun Group Inc.
Nisshin Sugar Mfg. Co., Ltd.
Novozymes Japan Ltd.
Ogawa & Co., Ltd.
Omron Healthcare Co., Ltd.
Otsuka Pharmaceutical Co., Ltd.
Procter & Gamble Far East Inc.
Rengo Co., Ltd.
Riken Vitamin Company, Ltd.
San-Ei Gen F.F.I., Inc.
Sankyo Co., Ltd.
Shin Mitsui Sugar Co., Ltd.
Shiratori Pharmaceutical
Company, Ltd.
Showa Sangyo Company, Ltd.
Snow Brand Milk Products
Co., Ltd.
Soda Aromatic Co., Ltd.
Sony Corporation
Sunny Health Co., Ltd.
Suntory Ltd.
Syngenta Seeds K.K.
T. Hasegawa Co., Ltd.
Taisho Pharmaceutical Co., Ltd.
Taiyo Kagaku Co., Ltd.

Takasago International
Corporation
Tanaka Foods Co., Ltd.
Teijin Pharma Ltd.
The Calpis Co., Ltd.
Tokyo Food Techno Co.
Towa Chemical Industry Co., Ltd.
Tsukishima Foods Industry
Co., Ltd.
Yakult Honsha Co., Ltd.
Yamazaki Baking Company, Ltd.

ILSI Korea

Coca-Cola Korea Co., Ltd.
Danisco Cultor
Doosan
International Flavors &
Fragrances (Korea) Inc.
Lotte Group R&D Center
Monsanto Korea Inc.
Roche Vitamins Korea Ltd.
VIXXOL Corporation

ILSI Mexico

American Quality Lab, S.A.
de C.V.
Arancia Corn Products, S.A. de
C.V.
Bimbo, S.A. de C.V.
Bristol-Myers Squibb de México
Coca-Cola/Servicios
Colloides Naturels de México, S.A.
de C.V.
Compañía Procter & Gamble de

México
Danisco Cultor, S.A. de C.V.
Grupo Warner Lambert, S. de R.L.
de C.V.
Kellogg de México, S.A. de C.V.
Masterfoods USA
Mazapanes Toledo, S.A. de C.V.
Monsanto Comercial, S.A. de C.V.
Nestlé México, S.A. de C.V.
Productos Kraft, S. de R.L. de C.V.
Roche Vitaminas México, S.A.
de C.V.
Sabritas, S. de R.L. de C.V.
Sensient Colors S.A. de C.V.
Unilever de México, S.A. de C.V.
Yakult, S.A. de C.V.

ILSI North Africa & Gulf Region

Atlantic Industries (Coca-Cola
Egypt)
The Egyptian Chamber of Food
Industries
Egyptian Company for Food
(Bisco Misr)
El-Nile Company for Food
Industries (ENJOY Company)
Kraft Foods Africa and Middle
East
Nestlé Egypt S.A.E.
Pepsi-Cola International Ltd.
Middle East and Africa Region
Procter & Gamble Egypt
Savola Sime Egypt Company

ILSI North America

3M Microbiology
Ajinomoto USA Inc.
Archer Daniels Midland Company
BASF Corporation
Cadbury Adams USA, LLC
Campbell Soup Company
Cargill, Incorporated
CNS, Inc.
The Coca-Cola Company
Colgate-Palmolive Company
ConAgra Foods
CTI Foods
Danisco USA, Inc.
DSM Nutritional Products Inc.
DuPont Haskell Laboratory
General Mills
Gerber Products Company
GlaxoSmithKline Research
H.J. Heinz Company
Hershey Foods Corporation
International Flavors &
Fragrances Inc.
Johnson & Johnson
Kellogg Company
Kraft Foods, Inc.
Masterfoods USA
McCormick & Company,
Incorporated
McNeil Nutritionals
Mead Johnson & Co.
Monsanto Company
National Starch and Chemical
Company
Nestlé USA, Inc.

Novozymes North America, Inc.
The NutraSweet Company
Nutrinova, Inc.
Ocean Spray Cranberries, Inc.
PepsiCo, Inc.
Pfizer, Inc.
The Procter & Gamble Company
Red Bull North America
Renessen LLC
Ross Products Division/Abbott
Laboratories
Sethness Products Company
Tate & Lyle North America
Unilever Bestfoods, North
America
Unilever Research USA
Wm. Wrigley Jr. Company

ILSI North Andean

Alimentos Kellogg S.A.
Alimentos Kraft de Colombia
Alpina Productos
Alimenticios S.A.
Amway Colombia
Cargill de Venezuela CA
Chicle Adams
Coca-Cola de Venezuela
Coca-Cola Servicios de
Colombia, S.A.
Colpromesa Promasa
Compañía Agrícola Colombiana
Compañía de Galletas Noel S.A.
Empresas Polar
Industrial Danec
Kellogg de Colombia

Kraft Food Ecuador
Meals de Colombia S.A.
Merisant Colombia S.A.
Moderna
Nestlé de Colombia
Nestlé del Ecuador
Nestlé Region Andina
Nestlé Venezuela
Parmalat Venezuela
Procter & Gamble de
Venezuela CA
PRONACA
Refreshment Product Services
Ecuador S.A. (Coca-Cola)
Sociedad Agrícola e Industrial San
Carlos
Unilever Bestfoods Greater
Andina S.A.
Unilever Ecuador
Yanbal Ecuador S.A.

ILSI South Africa

Coca-Cola Southern Africa
DSM Nutritional Products
Masterfoods South Africa
(Pty) Ltd.
Monsanto South Africa (Pty) Ltd.
Nampak Group
Nestlé South Africa
Pioneer Food Group Ltd.
Unilever Bestfoods Robertsons

ILSI South Andean

Alusud Embalajes Chile Ltda.

Coca-Cola de Chile S.A.
Córpora Tresmontes S.A.
DSM Nutritional Products
Chile S.A.
Envases CMF S.A.
Kellogg Chile Ltda.
McDonald's Chile S.A.
Monsanto Moviagro Chile S.A.
The Nutrasweet Company

ILSI Southeast Asia Region

Ajinomoto (Singapore) Pte. Ltd.
Ajinomoto Co., (Thailand) Ltd.
Akzo Nobel Chemicals Pte. Ltd.
Cerebos Pacific Limited
The Coca-Cola Export
Corporation
Danisco Sweeteners/Danisco
Australia Pty. Ltd.
DSM Nutritional Products Asia
Pacific Pte. Ltd.
The East Asiatic Company
(Singapore) Pte. Ltd.
Gerber Products Company/
Novartis Consumer Health, Inc.
Goodman Fielder Ltd.
Heinz Singapore Pte. Ltd.
International Flavors &
Fragrances Inc.
Kraft Foods, Limited
Mars Incorporated
Monsanto Company
Nestlé R&D Center (Pte) Ltd.
New Zealand Milk
The NutraSweet Company

Pepsi-Cola Limited
The Procter & Gamble Company
PT Indofood Sukses Makmur
PT Sinar Sosro
SIS'88 Pte. Ltd.
The Solae Company
Unilever Asia Pte. Ltd.
Yeo Hiap Seng Ltd.

http://www.ilsi.org/about/index.cfm?pubentityid=3#

Appendix V

FDA Final Rule Report Acesulfame K

Final Rule
http://www.fda.gov/OHRMS/DOCKETS/98fr/03-32101.
htm

Federal Register: December 31, 2003 (Volume 68, Number 250)
Rules and Regulations
Page 75411-75413
From the Federal Register Online via GPO Access [wais.access.gpo.gov]
DOCID: fr31de03-15

Department Of Health And Human Services

Food and Drug Administration
21 CFR Part 172
Docket No. 2002F-0220

Food Additives Permitted for Direct Addition to Food for Human Consumption; Acesulfame Potassium

AGENCY: Food and Drug Administration, HHS.

ACTION: Final rule.

SUMMARY: The Food and Drug Administration (FDA) is amending the food additive regulations to provide for the safe use of acesulfame potassium (ACK) as a general-purpose sweetener and flavor enhancer in food, not including meat and poultry.

This action[Page 75412] is in response to a food additive petition filed by Nutrinova, Inc. It will simplify the existing regulations by replacing all of the currently listed uses of ACK with a single-use category for food.

DATES: This rule is effective December 31, 2003. Submit written or electronic objections and requests for a hearing by January 30, 2004.

ADDRESSES: Submit written objections and requests for a hearing to the Division of Dockets Management (HFA-305), Food and Drug Administration, 5630 Fishers Lane, rm. 1061, Rockville, MD 20852. Submit electronic objections at http://frwebgate.access.gpo.gov/cgi-bin/leaving.cgi?from=leavingFR.html&log=linklog&to=http://www.fda.gov/dockets/ecomments.

FOR FURTHER INFORMATION CONTACT: Blondell Anderson, Center for Food Safety and Applied Nutrition (HFS-265), Food and Drug Administration, 5100 Paint Branch Pkwy., College Park, MD 20740-3835, 202-418-3106.

Supplementary Information:

I. Background

In a notice published in the Federal Register on May 20, 2002 (67 FR 35552), FDA announced that Nutrinova, Inc., 285 Davidson Ave., suite
102, Somerset, NJ 08873, had filed a food additive petition (FAP 2A4735). The petition proposed to amend Sec. 172.800 Acesulfame potassium (21 CFR 172.800) to provide for the safe use of ACK as a general-purpose sweetener and flavor enhancer.

ACK is currently approved under Sec.172.800 for use in 12 food categories at levels determined by current good manufacturing practice. The existing regulation has resulted from the approval of seven food additive petitions (FAPs). The practical effect of the amendment requested in the current petition would be to broaden the regulation to include any additional food category not allowed by the current regulation, with the exception, as discussed in the following paragraphs, of meat and poultry, and to replace the 12 currently listed uses of ACK with a single-use category for food.

The acceptable daily intake (ADI) of 15 milligrams per kilogram body weight per day (mg/kg bw/d) or 900 mg per person per day (mg/p/d) was established for ACK as a result of FDA's review of FAP 2A3659 (53 FR 28379, July 28, 1988), which resulted in the agency's initial approval of ACK in several food categories. The ADI is the level of consumption that has been determined to be safe for human consumption every day over an entire lifetime. The present petition does not contain any new information that would cause FDA to alter this previously determined ADI for ACK.

FDA's review of the petitions submitted subsequent to FAP 2A3659 involved primarily the following factors: (1) An assessment of the estimated exposure from each additional use; and (2) a determination of whether the cumulative estimated exposure, including the newly requested use, would cause the ADI for ACK to be exceeded over a lifetime by individuals who consume ACK at high levels. In its evaluation of ACK for use in nonalcoholic beverages, including beverage bases, FDA also assessed the safety from exposure to acetoacetamide-N-sulfonic acid (AAS) and acetoacetamide (AAA), the two principal hydrolysis products of ACK (63 FR 36344 at 36346 to 36355, July 6, 1998).

Although the functionality of ACK was addressed in earlier FAPs, in the current petition, Nutrinova, Inc., provided the results from taste panel studies demonstrating the sweetness profile of ACK as a function of concentration in a variety of foods. These data demonstrate that ACK can be used alone or in blends with other intense sweeteners or bulk sweeteners (e.g., sucrose) at self-limiting levels depending on the food application (Ref. 1).

II. Determination of Safety

Under the general safety standard provisions of section 409(c)(3)(A) of the Federal Food, Drug, and Cosmetic Act (the act) (21 U.S.C. 348(c)(3)(A)), a food additive cannot be approved for a particular use unless a fair evaluation of the data available to FDA establishes that the additive is safe for that use. FDA's food additive regulations (21 CFR 170.3(i)) define safe as a "reasonable certainty in the minds of competent scientists that the substance is not harmful under the intended conditions of use."

The food additives anticancer, or Delaney, clause (section 409(c)(3)(A) of the act) further provides that no food additive shall be deemed to be safe if it is found to induce cancer when ingested by man or animal. Importantly, however, the Delaney clause applies to the additive itself and not to constituents of the additive. Thus, where an additive has not been shown to cause cancer, even though it contains a carcinogenic impurity, the additive is not subject to the legal effect of the Delaney clause. Rather, the additive is properly evaluated under the general safety standard using risk assessment procedures to determine whether there is a reasonable certainty that no harm will result from the proposed use of the additive (Scott v. FDA, 728 F.2d 322 (6th Cir. 1984)).

III. Evaluation of Safety for the Petitioned Uses of the Food Additive

To determine whether ACK can be safely used as a general-purpose sweetener and flavor enhancer, FDA focused its evaluation on whether human exposure to ACK from these uses would exceed the ADI of 15 mg/kg bw/d, and on the potential health risk from exposure to the primary hydrolysis products, AAS and AAA, and the impurity, methylene chloride.

A. Exposure to ACK, AAS, and AAA

FDA has determined the cumulative estimated daily intake (CEDI) for ACK from its use as a general-purpose sweetener and flavor enhancer in food for eaters-only at the 90th percentile intake to be 313 mg/p/d (Refs. 2 and 3). This CEDI is based on the following factors: (1) The amount of ACK that may be used in the currently regulated food categories and (2) the maximum use level of ACK in other representative food categories in which the sweetener may be used. FDA concludes that the updated CEDI for ACK is well below the ADI (900 mg/p/d). FDA has determined that the updated CEDIs for AAS and AAA are 250 micrograms per person per day ([mu]g/p/day) and 0.36 [mu]g/p/day, respectively (Refs. 1 and 3). These hydrolysis products are formed only under extreme conditions of temperature and/or pH. The agency has determined that the increase in exposure to AAS and AAA, due to the additional uses, is negligible and does not pose any safety concerns (Refs. 3, 4, and 5).

B. Methylene Chloride

Methylene chloride, a carcinogenic chemical, is a potential impurity in ACK resulting from its use as a solvent in the initial manufacturing step of the sweetener. Data previously submitted in FAP 0A4212 show that methylene chloride could not be detected in the final product at a limit of detection (LOD) of

40 parts per billion (ppb) as discussed in the July 6, 1998, final rule (63 FR 36344 at 36346). In the past, FDA has assumed that methylene chloride is present in ACK at the LOD of 40 ppb (worst-case scenario) and has evaluated its safety by performing a risk assessment for methylene chloride based on this level. No new information has been received to change FDA's previous risk assessment for methylene chloride. Moreover, FDA does not expect that methylene chloride will be present in ACK due to the following [Page 75413] factors: (1) The multi-step purification process used in the manufacture of ACK and (2) the volatility of methylene chloride (Ref. 1).

IV. Conclusion

FDA has reviewed the information available in its files on ACK and its hydrolysis products, as well as the current petition, and concludes that there is a reasonable certainty that no harm will result from the use of ACK as a general-purpose sweetener and flavor enhancer in foods. However, in accordance with a memorandum of understanding between the Food Safety and Inspection Service (FSIS), United States Department of Agriculture, and FDA (65 FR 51758, August 25, 2000), a restriction from use "in meat and poultry" is included in the ACK regulation. This restriction is applied when the petitioner does not specify that the food additive is intended for such use. At this time, FSIS has not evaluated data on the suitability of use of ACK in meat or poultry. Therefore, FDA concludes that the food additive regulations should be amended as set forth in this document.

In accordance with Sec.171.1(h) (21 CFR 171.1(h)), the petition and the documents that FDA considered and relied upon in reaching its decision to approve the petition are available for inspection at the Center for Food Safety and Applied Nutrition by appointment with the information contact person. As provided in Sec. 171.1(h), FDA will delete from the documents any materials that are not available for public disclosure before making the documents available for inspection.

V. Environmental Effects

FDA has carefully considered the potential environmental effects of this action. FDA concluded that the action will not have a significant impact on the human environment, and that an environmental impact statement is not required. FDA's finding of no significant impact and the evidence supporting that finding, contained in an environmental assessment, may be seen in the Division of Dockets Management (see ADDRESSES) between 9 a.m. and 4 p.m., Monday through Friday.

VI. Paperwork Reduction Act of 1995

This final rule contains no collection of information. Therefore, clearance by the Office of Management and Budget under the Paperwork Reduction Act of 1995 is not required.

VII. Objections

Any person who will be adversely affected by this regulation may at any time file with the Division of Dockets Management (see ADDRESSES) written or electronic objections on or before January 30, 2004. Each objection shall be separately numbered, and each numbered objection shall specify with particularity the provisions of the regulation to which objection is made and the grounds for the objection. Each numbered objection on which a hearing is requested shall specifically so state. Failure to request a hearing for any particular objection shall constitute a waiver of the right to a hearing on that objection. Each numbered objection for which a hearing is requested shall include a detailed description and analysis of the specific factual information intended to be presented in support of the objection in the event that a hearing is held. Failure to include such a description and analysis for any particular objection shall constitute a waiver of the right to a hearing on the objection. Three copies of all documents shall be submitted and shall be identified with the docket number found in brackets in the heading of this document. Any objections received in response to the regulation may be seen in the Division of Dockets Management (see ADDRESSES) between 9 a.m. and 4 p.m., Monday through Friday.

VIII. References

The following references have been placed on display in the Division of Dockets Management (see ADDRESSES) and may be seen by interested persons between 9 a.m. and 4 p.m., Monday through Friday.

1. Memorandum from D. Robie, Division of Petition Review, Chemistry Review Group, to B. Anderson, Division of Petition Review, Regulatory Group II, October 7, 2002, and addendum memorandum from S. E. Carberry, Division of Petition Review, Chemistry Review Group, to B. Anderson, Division of Petition Review, Regulatory Group I, August 28, 2003.
2. Memorandum from D. Robie, Division of Petition Review, Chemistry Review Group to B. Anderson, Division of Petition Review, Regulatory Group II, March 19, 2003, and addendum memorandum from S. E. Carberry, Division of Petition Review, Chemistry Review Group, to B. Anderson, Division of Petition Review, Regulatory Group I, August 28, 2003.
3. Memorandum to the file, July 7, 2003.
4. Memorandum from M. Bleiberg, Division of Petition Review, Toxicology Review Group I, to B. Anderson, Division of Petition Review, Regulatory Group I, December 18, 2002.
5. Memorandum from M. Bleiberg, Division of Petition

Review, Toxicology Review Group I, to B. Anderson, Division of Petition Review, Regulatory Group II, April 2, 2003.

List of Subjects in 21 CFR Part 172 Food additives, Reporting and recordkeeping requirements.

Therefore, under the Federal Food, Drug, and Cosmetic Act and under authority delegated to the Commissioner of Food and Drugs, 21 CFR part 172 is amended as follows:

Part 172 - Food Additives Permitted For Direct Addition To Food For Human Consumption

1. The authority citation for 21 CFR Part 172 continues to read as follows: Authority: 21 U.S.C. 321, 341, 342, 348, 371, 379e.
2. Section 172.800 is amended by revising the introductory paragraph and paragraph (c), and by removing paragraphs (d) and (e) to read as follows:

Sec. 172.800 Acesulfame potassium.

Acesulfame potassium (CAS Reg. No. 55589-62-3), also known as acesulfame K, may be safely used as a general-purpose sweetener and flavor enhancer in foods generally, except in meat and poultry, in accordance with current good manufacturing practice and in an amount not to exceed that reasonably required to accomplish the intended technical effect in foods for which standards of identity established under section 401 of the Federal Food, Drug, and Cosmetic Act do not preclude such use, under the following conditions:

(a) * * *
(b) * * *
(c) If the food containing the additive is represented

to be for special dietary uses, it shall be labeled in compliance with part 105 of this chapter.

Dated: December 17, 2003.
Jeffrey Shuren,
Assistant Commissioner for Policy.

FR Doc. 03-32101 Filed 12-30-03; 8:45 am
BILLING CODE 4160-01-S

Appendix VI
FDA Final Rule Report Neotame

Patent Extension Request by The NutraSweet Company
Federal Register: July 7, 2004 (Volume 69, Number 129)
Notices Page 40946
From the Federal Register Online via GPO Access (wais.access.
gpo.gov) DOCID:fr07jy04-105

Department Of Health And Human Services

Food and Drug Administration
Docket No. 2003E-0257

Determination of Regulatory Review Period for Purposes of
Patent Extension; Neotame

AGENCY: Food and Drug Administration, HHS.

ACTION: Notice.

SUMMARY: The Food and Drug Administration (FDA)
has determined the regulatory review period for neotame and is
publishing this notice of that determination as required by law.
FDA has made the determination because of the submission
of an application to the Director of Patents and Trademarks,
Department of Commerce, for the extension of a patent which
claims that food additive.

ADDRESSES: Submit written comments and petitions to the
Division of Dockets Management (HFA-305), Food and Drug
Administration, 5630 Fishers Lane, rm. 1061, Rockville, MD

20852. Submit electronic comments to: http://frwebgate.access. gpo.gov/cgibin/leaving.cgi?from=leavingFR.html&log=linklog &to=http://www.fda.gov/dockets/ecomments.

FOR FURTHER INFORMATION CONTACT: Claudia Grillo, Office of Regulatory Policy (HFD-013), Food and Drug Administration, 5600 Fishers Lane, Rockville, MD 20857, 240-453-6699.

SUPPLEMENTARY INFORMATION: The Drug Price Competition and Patent Term Restoration Act of 1984 (Public Law 98-417) and the Generic Animal Drug and Patent Term Restoration Act (Public Law 100-670) generally provide that a patent may be extended for a period of up to 5 years so long as the patented item (human drug product, animal drug product, medical device, food additive, or color additive) was subject to regulatory review by FDA before the item was marketed. Under these acts, a product's regulatory review period forms the basis for determining the amount of extension an applicant may receive.

A regulatory review period consists of two periods of time: A testing phase and an approval phase. For food additives, the testing phase begins when a major health or environmental effects test involving the food additive begins and runs until the approval phase begins. The approval phase starts with the initial submission of a petition requesting the issuance of a regulation for use of the food additive and continues until FDA grants permission to market the food additive. Although only a portion of a regulatory review period may count toward the actual amount of extension that the Director of Patents and Trademarks may award (for example, half the testing phase must be subtracted as well as any time that may have occurred before the patent was issued), FDA's determination of the length of a regulatory review period for a food additive will include all of the testing phase and approval phase as specified in 35 U.S.C. 156(g)(2)(B).

Appendix VI – FDA Final Rule Report Neotame

FDA recently approved for marketing the food additive neotame. Neotame is a nonnutritive sweetener in food. Subsequent to this approval, the Patent and Trademark Office received a patent term restoration application for neotame (U.S. Patent No. 5,480,668) from The NutraSweet Co., and the Patent and Trademark Office requested FDA's assistance in determining this patent's eligibility for patent term restoration. In a letter dated July 16, 2003, FDA advised the Patent and Trademark Office that this food additive had undergone a regulatory review period and that the approval of neotame represented the first permitted commercial marketing or use of the product. Thereafter, the Patent and Trademark Office requested that FDA determine the product's regulatory review period.

FDA has determined that the applicable regulatory review period for neotame is 3,143 days. Of this time, 1,503 days occurred during the testing phase of the regulatory review period, 1,640 days occurred during the approval phase. These periods of time were derived from the following dates:

1. The date a major health or environmental effects test ("test") involving this food additive was begun: December 2, 1993. FDA has verified the applicant's claim that the test was begun on December 2, 1993.
2. The date the petition requesting the issuance of a regulation for use of the additive ("petition") was initially submitted with respect to the food additive under section 409 of the Federal Food, Drug and Cosmetic Act (21 U.S.C. 348): January 12, 1998. The applicant claims December 17, 1997, as the date the petition for neotame was initially submitted; however, FDA records indicate that the petition was submitted on January 12, 1998.
3. The date the petition became effective: July 9, 2002. FDA has verified the applicant's claim that

the regulation for the additive became effective/
commercial marketing was permitted on July 9, 2002.

This determination of the regulatory review period establishes
the maximum potential length of a patent extension. However,
the U.S. Patent and Trademark Office applies several statutory
limitations in its calculations of the actual period for patent
extension. In its application for patent extension, this applicant
seeks 973 days of patent term extension.

Anyone with knowledge that any of the dates as published are
incorrect may submit to the Division of Dockets Management
(see ADDRESSES) written or electronic comments and ask
for a redetermination by September 7, 2004. Furthermore,
any interested person may petition FDA for a determination
regarding whether the applicant for extension acted with due
diligence during the regulatory review period by January 3,
2005. To meet its burden, the petition must contain sufficient
facts to merit an FDA investigation. (See H. Rept. 857, part 1,
98th Cong., 2d sess., pp. 41-42, 1984.) Petitions should be in the
format specified in 21 CFR 10.30.

Comments and petitions should be submitted to the Division
of Dockets Management. Three copies of any mailed information
are to be submitted, except that individuals may submit one copy.
Comments are to be identified with the docket number found
in brackets in the heading of this document. Comments and
petitions may be seen in the Division of Dockets Management
between 9 a.m. and 4 p.m., Monday through Friday.

Dated: June 21, 2004.
Jane A. Axelrad, Associate Director for Policy, Center for Drug
Evaluation and Research. [FR Doc. 04-15275 Filed 7-6-04; 8:45
am]

BILLING CODE 4160-01-S

Appendix VII
Saccharin Final Rule Report of Safety

3357 Federal Register/ Vol. 69, No. 115 / Wednesday, June 16, 2004 / Rules and Regulations

Special Analyses

**27 CFR Parts 4, 5, and 7 [T.D. TTB–12] RIN 1513–AA93
Removal of Requirement To Disclose
Saccharin in the Labeling of Wine,
Distilled Spirits, and Malt Beverages (2003R–575P)
AGENCY:** Alcohol and Tobacco Tax and
Trade Bureau, Treasury. **ACTION:** Final rule; Treasury decision.

SUMMARY: This document amends the Alcohol and Tobacco Tax and Trade Bureau's labeling regulations to remove the requirement for bottlers of wine, distilled spirits, and malt beverages to show a warning on products containing saccharin. The regulatory amendments in this document reflect the National Toxicology Program's revised findings about saccharin and the removal of the statutory requirement for the warning.

DATES: This rule is effective on June 16, 2004.

FOR FURTHER INFORMATION CONTACT: Lisa M. Gesser, Regulations and Procedures Division, Alcohol and Tobacco Tax and Trade Bureau, P.O. Box 128, Morganza, Maryland 20660; (301–290–1460) or e- mail *Lisa.Gesser@ttb. gov.*

Supplementary Information:

Background

The Federal Alcohol Administration Act, 27 U.S.C. 205(e)(2), authorizes the Administrator of the Alcohol and Tobacco Tax and Trade Bureau (TTB), as a delegate of the Secretary of the Treasury, to prescribe regulations which will provide the consumer with "adequate information" as to the identity and quality of alcohol beverage products. Under this authority, parts 4,5, and 7 of title 27 of the Code of Federal Regulations (27 CFR 4, 5, and 7) prescribe the labeling requirements for wines, distilled spirits, and malt beverages, respectively. Prior to January 24, 2003, the Secretary of the Treasury had delegated this responsibility to the Administrator's predecessor, the Director of the former Bureau of Alcohol, Tobacco and Firearms, Department of the Treasury (ATF- Treasury). The regulations requiring basic mandatory labeling information for alcohol beverage products have been in effect for over 50 years. Decision ATF–220 on December 20, 1985 at 50 FR 51851 (as corrected in 51 FR 4338, published February 4, 1986). Treasury Decision ATF–220 amended the regulations in 27 CFR parts 4, 5, and 7 to require bottlers of alcohol beverage products containing saccharin (including sodium saccharin, calcium saccharin and ammonium saccharin) to label their products with a health warning statement identical to that set forth in the Saccharin Study and Labeling Act. On May 15, 2000, the U.S. Department of Health and Human Services, Public Health Service, National Toxicology Program published the 9th Report on Carcinogens. **The Report delisted saccharin, which had been listed in the Report as "reasonably anticipated to be a human carcinogen" since 1981.**

The Report explained that saccharin was removed from the list after a review of the carcinogenicity data for saccharin. The Report concluded: **Saccharin will be removed from the Report on Carcinogens, because the rodent cancer data are not**

sufficient to meet the current criteria to list this chemical as *reasonably anticipated to be a human carcinogen*. This is based on the perception that the observed bladder tumors in rats arise by mechanisms not relevant to humans, and the lack of data in humans suggesting a carcinogenic hazard. Section 517, Title V, Appendix A, Consolidated Appropriations Act of 2001 (Pub. L. 106–554, 114 Stat. 2763), repealed 21 U.S.C. 343(o), the saccharin warning statement requirement, as well as subsections (c) and (d) of section 4 of the Saccharin Study and Labeling Act. Accordingly, we are amending 27 CFR parts 4, 5, and 7 by removing the saccharin warning statement requirement for the labeling of wine, distilled spirits, and malt beverages. These regulatory changes are made solely to reflect the statutory change noted above, and are in no way intended to reflect or prejudice our review of a recent petition we have received, proposing a number of new and broader labeling requirements.

Executive Order 12866

On November 23, 1977, President Carter signed into law the Saccharin Study and Labeling Act, Public Law 95– 203, 91 Stat. 1451. Section 4(a)(1) of the Saccharin Study and Labeling Act added Paragraph (o) to 21 U.S.C. 343, requiring the Following statement on the labels of all food and beverage products that contained saccharin:

Use of this product may be hazardous to your health. This product contains saccharin, which has been determined to cause cancer in laboratory animals.

In 1984 and 1985, ATF-Treasury began receiving petitions from industry members requesting to use saccharin as a sugar substitute in alcohol beverage manufacturing. The Food and Drug Administration regulations, 21 CFR 180.37 (21 U.S.C. 348, 371), did not and still do not prevent the use of saccharin in the production of alcohol beverages in recognition of the

Congressional mandate as expressed in the Saccharin Study and Labeling Act and pursuant to section 205(e)(2) of the Federal Alcohol Administration Act, ATF-Treasury published Treasury.

Appendix VIII

European Commission's Report on Sucralose

European Commission Health & Consumer Protection Directorate-General

Directorate C - Scientific Opinions

Scientific Committee On Food Scf/Cs/Adds/Edul/190 Final

12/9/2000

Opinion of the Scientific Committee on Food on sucralose (Adopted by the SCF on September 7, 2000)

For the full text report and Annex I, visit http://www.splendaexposed.com.

Annex 2: Studies Submitted On Sucralose

Study	NOEL mg/kg	LOEL mg/kg	Effects
Acute oral toxicity in mice	>16000		
Acute oral toxicity in rats	>10000		
4-8 week dietary study in rats	500	1250 2500	↓ female bw gain, ↓ female & male bw gain, ↓ spleen wt, ↓ thymus wt and cellular changes
26-week dietary administration and dietary restriction in rats	628-787	1973-2455	↓ Bw gain, ↓ food intake
12-month dietary study in dogs	>874		Highest dose NOEL
Teratology oral gavage study in rats	>2000		Highest dose NOEL
Teratology oral gavage study in rabbits	350	700	Maternal gastro-intestinal effects
Teratology oral gavage range-finding study in rabbits	900		
Teratology oral gavage study in rabbits	350	1000	Maternal gastro-intestinal effects
Two-generation dietary reproduction study in rats	Not established	150	↓ Bw gain, ↓ food intake
2-year dietary chronic toxicity/ carcinogenicity study in mice	1500	4500	↓ Bw, ↑ Liver wt, ↓ erythrocytes, nephropathy
2-year dietary chronic toxicity/ carcinogenicity study in rats with in utero exposure	Not established	150	↓ Bw gain, ↓ food intake

Appendix VIII – European Commission's Report on Sucralose

Study	NOEL mg/kg	LOEL mg/kg	Effects
Mineral bioavailability with dietary administration in rats	1000	2000	↓ Bw gain, ↓ food intake, ↑ caecal wt
21-day oral gavage neurotoxicity study in mice	>1000		Highest dose NOEL
4- to 13-week oral gavage study in rats	Not established	2000	↑ Bw gain, ↑ food intake, ↑ kidney wt, ↓ spleen wt, variable thymus wt
26-week oral gavage study in rats	1500	3000	↓ bw gain, ↑ caecal wt
28-day Tier I oral immunotoxicity in rats by oral gavage and diet	1500	3000	↓ Bw gain
Gene mutation in bacteria			Negative
Gene mutation in mammalian cells in vitro (mouse lymphoma assay)			Negative
Chromosome aberrat ions in human lymphocytes in vitro			Negative
In vivo rat bone marrow cytogenetics			Negative
Mouse micronucleus test			Negative
Absorption, distribution, metabolism and excretion in rat, dog and man, and metabolism in rabbit			
Pharmacokinetics after oral administration to pregnant rats and rabbits			
Comparative pharmacokinetics, dietary and oral gavage administration in rats			
8-week palatability study in rats			

Splenda® *Is It Safe Or Not?*

Study	NOEL mg/kg	LOEL mg/kg	Effects
Acceptability in diet in rats			
Acceptability in water in rats			
Glycolysis in various rat tissues in vitro			
Insulin secretion in rats in vivo			
Glycolytic activity of rat sperm			
Liver enzyme induction in rats			
Short-term clinical study in normal human volunteers			See Annex 1
13-week clinical study in normal human volunteers			See Annex 1
Insulin secret ion and sucrose absorption in normal human volunteers			See Annex 1
Glycaemic effect of a single high oral dose in diabetic patients			See Annex 1
6-month study of glucose homeostasis in non-insulin-dependent diabetes			See Annex 1
Specific clinical chemistry parameters in 6-month study of glucose in non- insulin-dependent diabetes			See Annex 1
12-week study of glucose homeostasis in normal volunteers			See Annex 1
3-month study of glucose homeostasis in non-insulin-dependent diabetes			See Annex 1

Annex 3: Studies submitted on hydrolysis products of sucralose, 4-CG and 1,6-DCF

Absorption, distribution metabolism and excretion in rats

Acute toxicity in mice and rats

Gene mutation in bacteria (S. typhimurium)

Gene mutation in mammalian cells in vitro (mouse lymphoma assay)

Chromosome aberrations in mammalian cells in vitro (human lymphocytes)

In vivo rat bone marrow cytogenetics

Dominant lethal mutations in mice

Sex-linked recessive lethal mutations in Drosophila melanogaster (1,6-DCF only)

In vivo sister chromatid exchange in the mouse (1,6-DCF only)

In vivo mouse micronucleus test (1,6-DCF only)

Covalent binding to DNA in vivo in rats (1,6-DCF only)

In vitro unscheduled DNA synthesis in rat hepatocytes (1,6-DCF only)

Teratogenicity in rats

Two-generation reproduction study in rats

Rat 2-year chronic toxicity/carcinogenicity study

90-day dietary study in rats

6-month dietary study in the dog

Appendix IX
Emergency Procedures for Chlorine

The Potential Hazards of Chlorine

Health hazards:

1. Poisonous; may be fatal if inhaled.
2. Contact may cause burns to skin and eyes.
3. Contact with liquid may cause frostbite.
4. Runoff from fire control or dilution water may cause pollution.

Fire or Explosion:

1. May ignite other combustible materials (wood, paper, oil, etc.).
2. Mixture with fuels may explode.
3. Cylinder may explode in heat of fire. Vapor explosion and poison hazard indoors, outdoors and in sewers.

Emergency Action:

Keep unnecessary people away; isolate hazard area and deny entry. Stay upwind, out of low areas, and ventilate closed spaces before entering. Positive pressure self-contained breathing apparatus (SCBA) and chemical protective clothing which is specifically OSHA recommend by the shipper or manufacturer may be worn. It may provide little or no thermal protection. Structural firefighters' protective clothing is **NOT** effective for these materials. Isolate the leak or spill area immediately for at least 150 feet in all directions. If you find the ID number and the name of the material there, begin protective action.

   CALL CHEMTREC AT 1-800-424-9300 FOR EMERGENCY ASSISTANCE. If water pollution occurs, notify the appropriate authorities.

First Aid:

1. Move victim to fresh air and call emergency medical care; if not breathing, give artificial respiration; if breathing is difficult, give oxygen.
2. In case of contact with material, immediately flush skin or eyes with running water for at least fifteen minutes.
3. Remove and isolate contaminated clothing and shoes at the site.
4. Keep victim quiet and maintain normal body temperature.
5. Effects may be delayed; keep victim under observation.

Fire:

Small Fires: <u>Water Only</u>:

1. No dry chemical, CO2 or halon.
2. Contain and let burn.
3. If fire must be fought, water or fog is recommended.
4. Move container from fire area if you can do it without risk.
5. Apply cooling water to sides of containers that are exposed to flames until well after fire is out.
6. Stay away from ends of tanks.
7. For massive fire in cargo area, use unmanned hose holder or monitor nozzles; if this is impossible, withdraw from area and let fire burn.

Appendix IX – Emergency Procedures for Chlorine

Spill Or Leak:

1. Keep combustibles (wood, paper, oil, etc.) away from spilled material.
2. Fully-encapsulating, vapor-protective clothing should be worn for spills and leaks with no fire.
3. Stop leak if you can do it without risk.
4. Water spray may be used to reduce or direct vapors.
5. Isolate area until gas has dispersed.

References
References and Sources of Additional Information

Chapter 1
Splenda: *Is It Safe Or Not?*

Bellin J. New Scientist. pg 13. Nov 23, 1991.

Federal Register. Vol. 63. No. 64. Rules and Regulations 16417-16433. Friday. April 3, 1998.

Patent info: http://www.cas.org/motw/sucrapub2.html

European Commission. Health & Consumer Protection Directorate-General. Opinion of the Scientific Committee on Food on sucralose. 7 September 2000. P.2.

Chlorine facts: http://www.bidness.com/esd/cl2facts.htm

Mattes RD, The taste for salt in humans. American Journal of Clinical Nutrition. Vol 65. 692S-697S. 1997.

Sacks, FM, et.al. Effects on Blood Pressure of Reduced Dietary Sodium and the Dietary Approaches to Stop Hypertension. DASH Diet. New England Journal of Medicine. Vol. 344. No. 1. January 4, 2001.

SRI Consulting (SRIC). PEP Review 90-1-4 Sucralose - A High Intensity, Noncaloric Sweetener. http://pep.sric.sri.com/Public/Reports/Phase_90/RW90-1-4/RW90-1-4.html

The Chemical Abstracts Service Registry number for sucralose: 56038-13-2.

Hydrolysis of sugars: the hydrolysis of sugar polymers by acid or enzymes converts non-reducing polysaccharides to reducing oligo- and monosaccharides. Biochemistry 2344 Lecture 11: Carbohydrates, March 29-April 2, 1999.

The Chemical Abstracts Service Registry number for sucralose: 56038-13-2.

Keith JN. Report 2.1460. Gastroenterology Section, AMB S401F (MC 4080): 188-1477. jnewton@medicine.bsd.uchicago.edu.

Hull JS. Sweet Poison: How The World's Most Popular Artificial Sweetener Is Killing Us-My Story. New Horizon Press, 1997.

Barndt R. L., & Jackson, G. (1990). Stability of sucralose in baked goods. *Food Technology, 44*, 62-66.

Wolraich ML, Hannah JN, Pinnock TY, Baumgaertel AI, Brown J. Comparison of diagnostic criteria for attention-deficit hyperactivity disorder in a county-wide sample. Journal of the American Academy of Child and Adolescent Psychiatry. 35 319-324, 1996.

Additional Resources

Grant D.L. Toxicological Evaluation. Division Health and Welfare Canada. For the entire research report, visit the following link: http://europa.eu.int/comm/food/fs/sc/scf/out68_en.pdf

Cyclamate Update: http://www.fda.gov/bbs/topics/ANSWERS/ANS00155.html

References

McCormick B. Doubts about aspartame. chicagotribune.com. Murray, 2004.04.14. http://groups.yahoo.com/group/aspartameNM/message/1104

Doi M, See H. Introduction to Polymer Physics. Oxford University Press, 1996.

Generalized Reaction of Dehydration Synthesis and Hydrolysis: dehydration synthesis and hydrolysis are reversible glucose + fructose sucrose + H 2 O. Physiological Effects and Case Studies. North Harris College Biology. http://science.nhmccd. edu/biol/dehydrat/dehydrat.html.

Harrison's Principles of Internal Medicine. RC 46.H333, 2001.

Current Medical Diagnosis and Treatment. RC 71.A14, 2004.

Merck Manual of Diagnosis and Therapy. RC 55.M4, 1999.

Wiggins JG. Comparing Standards of Mental Health Care: combined psychotherapy/pharmacotherapy vs. usual medical services. Paper presented, September, 1994.

McCormick B. Special to the Tribune. Chicago Tribune. pg. 9, Jul 14, 2004. http://www.chicagotribune.com/features/food/chi-0407140042jul14,1,4705778.story?coll=chi-homepagenews2-utl.

Young LR, Nestle M J. Estimating serving size. American Dietetics Assn. 98:458-59, 1998.

Children's Defense Fund. CMHS. Mental Health, USA, 1994.

National Mental Health Association. Mental Health Information and Statistics, March, 1997. http://www.

mhsource.com/resource/mh.html

Department of Microbiology. Colorado State University. Fort Collins, CO 80523.

Garcia A, Mount JR, Davidson PM. Ozone and Chlorine Treatment of Minimally Processed Lettuce. Jul 21, 2004.

Renwick AG. The metabolism of intense sweeteners. Xenobiotica. (10-11):1057-71. Review. Oct-Nov 16, 1986.

CHADD. Fact Sheet No. 3. Evidence-based Medication Management for Children and Adolescents with AD/HD.

Sulfuryl chloride, SO2Cl2: a highly reactive gaseous compound. DOC 508/877-8723, 1983. www.tylerbosmeny.com/ChemFiles/equilibrium.doc

Utz J. What Percentage of Your Body Is Water? Neuroscience Pediatrics. Allegheny University. May 15, 2000.

Bertino M, Beauchamp GK, Engelman K. Long-term reduction in dietary sodium alters the taste of salt. American Journal of Clinical Nutrition. Vol 36. 1134-1144. 1982.

Other Chemical Sweeteners

Amine The MSDS HyperGlossary. www.ilpi.com/msds/ref/amine.html

Blaylock RL. Connection between MS and aspartame. http://www.russellblaylockmd.com/

Cyclamate. http://www.fangda.com.hk/english/

Ophardt CE. Virtual Chembook: cyclamate. Elmhurst College.

References

http://www.ncbi.nlm.nih.gov/entrez/query.fcgi?CMD=Search &DB=pubmed

Hull JS. Sweet Poison: How The World's Most Popular Artificial Sweetener Is Killing Us-My Story. New Horizon Press, 1997.

Mukhopadhyay M, Mukherjee A, Chakrabarti J. In vivo cytogenetic studies on blends of aspartame and acesulfame-K. Food Chem Toxicol. 38(1): 75-7. Jan, 2000.

Ilback NG, Alzin M, Jahrl S, Enghardt-Barbieri H, Busk L. Estimated intake of the artificial sweeteners acesulfame-K, aspartame, cyclamate and saccharin in a group of Swedish diabetics, Food Addit Contam. 20 (2):99-114. PMID: 12623659. Feb, 2003.

Renwick AG. Acceptable daily intake and the regulation of intense sweeteners. Review. Food Addit Contam. 7 (4):463-75. Jul-Aug, 1990.

Hughes AM, Everitt BJ, Herbert J. The effects of simultaneous or separate infusions of some pro-opiomelanocortin-derived peptides (beta-endorphin, melanocyte stimulating hormone, and corticotrophin-like intermediate polypeptide) and their acetylated derivatives upon sexual and ingestive behaviour of male rats. Neuroscience. 27 (2): 689-98. Nov, 1988.

Chapter 2
Chlorine: In Your Swimming Pool And In Your Diet Cola

OLSWANG. Law Offices: representatives for Tate & Lyle plc. London. WC1V 6XX. 2. pg 1. August 20, 2004.

Emergency Response Guidebook: guidebook for first response to hazardous materials incidents. US Department of Transportation. DOT P 5800.5. 2000.

Maryland Sea Grant College Program. Maryland Program Directory Sea Grant. http://www.mdsg.umd.edu/PROGDIR.PDF

Chlorine Online Information Resource. Chlorine Industry Review Annual report: European chlorine industry update on economic, environmental and regulatory aspects, including statistical data on chlorine production and use. 2002-2003. http://www.eurochlor.org/chlorine/publications/publications.htm

Chlorine/Chloramine. The dangers of chlorine and chloramine in your tap water, and how to remove the danger. Natural Aquariums. Long Island Business News. http://www.csd.net/~cgadd/aqua/index.htm

Vallentyne J. Senior Scientist. What are Organochlorines and why are they so dangerous? Canada Centre for Inland Waters. Burlington, Ontario, http://webhome.idirect.com/~born2luv/backgrounder.html

Occupational and Environmental Medicine. 385-394. June 2003. http://oem.bmjjournals.com/cgi/content/full/60/6/385

References

Ledger J. The Environmental Impact Of Swimming Pools. African Wildlife. Issue 57. No. 2, Autumn, 2003 (Apr/May/Jun).

Environmental Health News. Occupational and Environmental Medicine. 385-394. The Association of State and Territorial Health Officials June 2003. http://oem.bmjjournals.com/cgi/content/full/60/6/385 and http://www.astho.org/pubs/June2003Newsletter.htm

Magnus P. Chlorinated Tap Water and Birth Defects. Paper presentation. Spina Bifida and Hydrocephalus Association. Feb 2000. http://www.lfsn.org/chlorina.htm

Thornton J, Halle M. Chlorinated tap water linked to birth defects. The Electronic Telegraph. London, England. February 20, 2000. http://www.telegraph.co.uk/portal/main.jhtml;sessionid=CIX0OQUEHPNJJQFIQMGSM54AVCBQWJVC?view=HOME&grid=P13&menuId=-1&menuItemId=-1&_requestid=116133

Chlorinated Water and Health Effects. Health Canada. November 4, 1998. http://www.hc-sc.gc.ca/ehp/ehd/bch/water_quality/chlorinated_water.htm

EPA Toxic Inventory Report on Phosgene: http://www.truthaboutsplenda.com/resources/links.html

Carson R. Silent Spring. 40th Anniversary Edition. Boston. Houghton Mifflin Company, 2002. http://www.rachelcarson.org/

Williamson J. Chlorine is a chemical whose time has passed: persistent organic pollutants (POPs) threaten the health and well-being of humans and wildlife. Chlorine Quandary. 2001 popularmechanics.com/science/research/2001/1/chlorine_ ban/print.phtml

Examining the Endocrine Question. discoveryhealth.com. November 15, 2004. http://health.discovery.com/premiers/toxic/inside.html

Van Bavel LB, Lindström GH, Carlberg M, Dreifaldt AC, Wijkström H, Starkhammar H, Eriksson M, Hallquist A, Kolmert T. Increased Concentrations of Polychlorinated Biphenyls, Hexachlorobenzene and Chlordanes in Mothers to Men with Testicular Cancer. Environmental Health Perspectives. 111 doi:10.1289/ehp.5816, 2003. http://www.ourstolenfuture.org/NewScience/reproduction/TDS/2003/2003-0115hardelletal.htm

Ames BN, Gold LS. Another perspective ...Nature's way. Consumer's Research Magazine. Vol. 76. No. 8. p. 20. August 1993.

DeGregori TR. Rockwell Lecture. Counter to Conventional Wisdom: In Defense of DDT and Against Chemophobia. Department of Economics. University of Houston. August 26, 1998. http://www.uh.edu/~trdegreg/ROCKWELL.HTM

Sienko MJ, Plane RA. Chemistry: Principles and Properties. McGraw-Hill. NY. 1966.

Williamson J. Chlorine is a chemical whose time has passed: persistent organic pollutants (POPs) threaten the health and well-being of humans and wildlife. Chlorine Quandary. 2001. http://www.popularmechanics.com/science/research/2001/1/chlorine_ban/print.phtml

Buccini B. Presentation. Intergovernmental Negotiating Committee. UNEP global POPs Convention. Johannesburg. 2000.

References

http://www.ourplanet.com/imgversn/124/buccini.html

CDC. Emergency Preparedness & Response. Medical Management Guidelines (MMGs) for Chlorine. Agency for Toxic Substances & Disease Registry. http://www.atsdr.cdc.gov/MHMI/mmg172.html

Chlorine Chemistry Council. Arlington, VA. http://c3.org/about_ccc/index.html

Burge D, Uhland V. Natural swimming pools. MotherEarthNews.com. http://www.motherearthnews.com/rec/hb/2075/

Environmentally safe mixtures.. Biodegradable ingredient cleaners. http://www.inlandtech.com

Additional Resources

Carr M. Flush with drugs. The Dallas Morning News. August, 2000.

Carr M. Prescription drugs turn up again in New Mexico rivers. The Dallas Morning News. AP Press. Jan. 21, 2001.

Chlorine and caustic soda. http://www.eurochlor.org/chlorine/publications/publications.htm

Chloramine Complications. Environmental Science & Technology. Science News. August 18, 2004.

Hays SM, Aylward LL. Dioxin risks in perspective: past, present, and future. Regulatory Toxicology and Pharmacology. 37. pp. 202-17. 2003.

Stop the Whitewash and the Waste: a project of the WEED Foundation. Contact:: 736 Bathurst Street. Toronto, Ontario. M5S 2R4. Phone: (416)5166-2600. Fax: (416)531-6214.

Armstrong L, Scott A. Whitewash: exposing the health and environmental dangers of women's sanitary products and disposable diapers -what you can do about it. Soft-cover. 196 pages. HarperCollins.

Johnson CM, Otolaryngol Head Neck Surgeon. Disposable plastic diapers: a foreign body hazard. 94 (2):235-6, 3d. Otolaryngologists and pediatricians should be aware of the potential hazard when examining diapered children with chronic rhinorrhea or sudden respiratory distress. PMID: 3083340. UI: 86176215. Feb, 1986.

Karlberg AT, Magnusson K. Rosin components identified in diapers. Contact Dermatitis. Division of Occupational Dermatology, National Institute of Occupational Health. Solna, Sweden. PMID: 8833460, UI: 96430334. Mar, 34 (3): 176-8O.

Additional research on DDT

Abelson PH. Chemicals: Perceptions versus facts. p.183. Science. Vol. 264. No. 5156. April 8, 1994.

Federal Register. Vol. 63. No. 64. Rules and Regulations 16417-16433. Friday. April 3, 1998.

Ames BN. Pollution, pesticides and cancer. pp.1-5. Journal of AOAC International. Vol. 75. 1992.

Ames B, Magaw R, Swirsky GL. Ranking possible carcinogenic hazards. pp. 76-92. Glickman and Gough eds. 1990.

References

Ames B, Profet M, Swirsky GL. Dietary pesticides (99.9% all natural). pp. 7777-7781. Proceedings of the National Academy of Sciences USA. Vol. 87. 1990.

Graham JD, Wiener JB. Risk vs. risk: tradeoffs in protecting health and the environment. Cambridge, MA. Harvard University Press. 1997.

Wakeford T. A Green in the machine. New Scientist. Vol. 132. No. 1743. November 2, 1991.

WHO (World Health Organization). DDT and its derivatives published under the joint sponsorship of the United Nations Environment Programme and the World Health Organization. Environmental health criteria 9. WHO Task Group on Environmental Health Criteria for DDT and its Derivatives. Geneva: World Health Organization. 1979.

WHO (World Health Organization). Health and sustainable development: 5 years after the earth summit. Geneva: Press Release WHO/47. June 18, 1997.

WRI (World Resources Institute). World resources 1998-99: a guide to the global environment: people and the environment: environmental change and human health. New York. Oxford University Press. 1998.

WWF (World Wide Fund for Nature). Time to ban DDT in Africa, says WWF. Electronic Mail & Guardian. June 30, 1998.

Hays SM, Aylward LL. Dioxin risks in perspective: past, present, and future. Regulatory Toxicology and Pharmacology. 37. 2003.

Additional U.S. Environmental Protection Agency (EPA) Reports: Pesticides. Chlorine Dioxide. http://www.epa.gov/pesticides/factsheets/chemicals/chlorinedioxidefactsheet.htm

Appendix B: summaries of environmental labeling. Report B-115. The Chlorine Free Products Association (CFPA). http://www.epa.gov/opptintr/epp/pubs/envlab/chlorine.pdf

EPA Clarifies Chlorine Production. MACT Regs. http://enviro.blr.com/display.cfm/id/41280

EPA Clarifies Chlorine Production MACT Regulations (ChemAlliance). EPA Clarifies Chlorine Production MACT Regulations. related links: http://www.chemalliance.org/News/news_detail.asp

Registry. Joint Food and Agriculture Organization/World Health Organization Expert Committee on Food Additives. The European Commission Scientific Committee on Food, and the U.S. Agency for Toxic Substances and Disease.

National Center for Environmental Health Publication. No. 02-0716. Second National Report on Human Exposure to Environmental Chemicals. *TEQ (toxic equivalent) is a quantitative measure of the combined toxicity of a mixture of dioxin-like chemicals. U.S. Centers for Disease Control and Prevention. 2003.

Chapter 3
Splenda Product List

http://www.splenda.com
http://www.splenda.com/page.jhtml?id=splenda/products/prodwithsplenda.inc

References

Chapter 4
Healthy Alternatives

Hull JS. Sweet Poison: How The World's Most Popular Artificial Sweetener Is Killing Us-My Story. New Horizon Press, 1997.

Horne J, Lawless HT, Speirs W, Sposato D.　Bitter taste of saccharin and acesulfame-K. Chem Senses. 27(1):31-8. Jan, 2002.

Report. The Joint Food and Agriculture Organization/World Health Organization Expert Committee on Food Additives (JECFA).

0-.alpha.-D-glucopyranosyl-D-sorbitol (1,1-GPS), mannitol, sorbitol, hydrogenated or non-hydrogenated oligosaccharides. www.pharmcast.com/Patents/Yr2002/April2002/041602/6372271_Chewing041602.htm

Stevia and Stevioside. Foods Stands Agency. March 27, 2002. http://www.food.gov.uk/multimedia/webpage/stevia

Stevia toxicity. http://www.Pubmed.com

http://wilstar.com/lowcarb/sugaralcohols.htm

Department of Health & Human Services. http://www.ncbi.nlm.nih.gov/entrez/query.fcgi?CMD=Search&DB=pubmed

Xylitol. http://www.xylipro.com/faq.html

Mung bean. http://www.sproutpeople.com/seed/mung.html

http://www.ethnohealth.com/eng/yac/yacintro.htm

http://medherb.com/92INULIN.HTM

Chapter 5
How To Eliminate Toxic Chemicals From Your Body

Hull JS. Sweet Poison: How The World's Most Popular Artificial Sweetener Is Killing Us-My Story. New Horizon Press, 1997.

Blaylock RL. Connection between MS and aspartame. http://www.russellblaylockmd.com/

Hull JS. Ten Steps To Detoxification: How To Cleanse Toxic Chemicals From Your Body. The Pickle Press, 2004.

Tate DF. Dieting study first to examine the use of information technology to aid weight loss. Journal of the American Medical Association, March 7, 2001.

Emery C. Exercise helps keep aging brains sharp. The Associated Press, April 27, 2004.

Pitchford P. Healing With Whole Foods: Oriental Traditions and Modern Nutrition. North Atlantic Books, 1993.

Ibid. pp. 214-215.

Chapter 6
Dying To Be Thin – Obesity And Diet Sweeteners

Van Wymelbeke V, Beridot-Therond ME, de La Gueronniere V, Fantino M., Eur J Clin Nutr., Jan; 58(1):154-61, 2004, "Influence of repeated consumption of beverages containing sucrose or intense sweeteners on food intake", National Library of Medicine, http://www.ncbi.nlm.nih.gov/entrez/query.fcgi?cmd=Retrieve&db=pubmed&dopt=Abstract&list_uids=14679381

References

"Portions Matter Nutrition Tips for Optimal Health", Dr. Kristine Clark, RD Director of Sports Nutrition, Pennsylvania State University.

Barbara Rippel, "How Food Standards Are Approved", *Consumers' Research Magazine*, Consumer Alert Column, April 2001.

International Food Standard Organization Faces Challenges, http://www.consumeralert.org/pubs/research/

Rolls BJ. Effects of intense sweeteners on hunger, food intake, and body weight: a review. Am J Clin Nutr. 1991 Apr; 53 (4):872-8.

Hull JS. Sweet Poison: How The World's Most Popular Artificial Sweetener Is Killing Us-My Story. New Horizon Press, 1997.

Constitution of the Advertising Standards Complaints Board. DECISION. Special Meeting 20 June 2005. Complaint 05/147 AWAP 05/5.

SWEET CHOICES: Questions & Answers about Sweeteners in Low-Calorie Foods and Beverages, http://www.caloriecontrol.org/benefit.html

THE OBESITY CRISIS: *Perils of portion distortion. Why Americans don't know when enough is enough.* Kim Severson, San Francisco Chronicle, March 2, 2004.

Blundell J.E., and Hill, A.J. Paradoxical effects of an intense sweetener (aspartame) on appetite. Lancet: 1092-1093, 1986.

Teff K.L., Devine, J., and Engelman, K., Sweet taste: effect on cephalic phase insulin release in men, Physiol Behavior 57:

1089-95, 1995.

Tordoff Michael G., Physiology and Behavior, 47: 555-559, 1990.

Ellington Darden, PhD, <u>A Flat Stomach ASAP</u>, Pocket Books, 1998.

http://www.bbc.co.uk/health/yourweight/whatis_stats.shtml

National Health and Nutrition Examination Survey (NHANES), http://www.niddk.nih.gov/health/nutrit/pubs/statobes.htm#what

BMJ USA: Editorial, "School soft drink intervention study. Too good to be true?" BMJ 2004;329:E315-E316 (14 August), doi:10.1136/bmj.329.7462.E315 http://bmj.bmjjournals.com/cgi/collection/obesity

Caballero B, Clay T, Davis SM, Ethelbah, B, et al., Pathways: a school-based, randomized controlled trial for the prevention of obesity in American Indian schoolchildren, Am J Clin Nutr 2003;78: 1030-1038.

Luepker RV, Perry CL, McKinlay SM, Nader PR, et al., Outcomes of a field trial to improve children's dietary patterns and physical activity. The Child and Adolescent Trial for Cardiovascular Health. CATCH collaborative group. JAMA 1996;275: 768-776.

Rockett HR, Colditz GA., Assessing diets of children and adolescents., Am J Clin Nutr 1997;65(4 suppl): 1116s-1122s.

Murray DM., Design and analysis of group-randomized trials. New York: Oxford University Press, 1998.

References

American Academy of Pediatrics Committee on School Health. Soft drinks in schools, Pediatrics 2004;113: 152-154.

Prevalence of Overweight Among Children and Adolescents: United States, 1999-2002, Results from the 1999-2002 National Health and Nutrition Examination Survey (NHANES), http://www.cdc.gov/nchs/products/pubs/pubd/hestats/overwght99.htm

Chapter 7
Artificial Sweetener Case Histories

Hull JS. Case histories. http://www.janethull.com

Hull JS. Case histories. http://www.sweetpoison.com

Hull JS. http://www.splendaexposed.com

Chapter 8
Research Studies

1. Federal Register. Vol. 63. No. 64. Rules and Regulations 16417-16433. Friday. April 3, 1998.

2. Gold M. http://www.holisticmed.com/splenda/

3. Bellin J. New Scientist. pg 13. Nov 23, 1991.

4. Knight L. Hydrophobic bonding of highly intense sweeteners. Deutsch and Hansch. *Pharmacology, 72,* 435-439. REVIEW. 1994.

5. Knight L. Kier. 1972.

6. Knight L. The development and applications of sucralose, a new high-intensity sweetener. Canadian Journal

of Physiology and Pharmacology. pg. 72. 435-439.
REVIEW, 1993.

7. Knight L. Wiet and Miller. 1997.

8. Ibid.

9. Van Wymelbeke V, Beridot-Therond ME, de La
   Gueronniere V, Fantino M. Universite de Bourgogne.
   Dijon, France.

10. Rats fed sweetener, not sugar, consume more calories.
    Purdue University. International Journal of Obesity. July
    8, 2004.

11. Ibid.

12. Health Canada. It's Your Health: Dioxins and Furans.
    The Health Effects of Dioxins and Furans. Jul 26, 2004.
    http://www.hc-sc.gc.ca/english/iyh/environment/
    dioxins.html

13. Ibid.

14. Ibid.

15. Federal Register. Vol. 63. No. 64. Rules and Regulations
    16417-16433. Friday. April 3, 1998.

16. Grice HC, Goldsmith LA. Sucralose - an overview of the
    toxicity data. Food Chemical Toxicology. 38. Supplement
    2. S1-S6, 2000.

17. Baird IM, Shephard NW, Merritt RJ, Hildick-Smith
    G. Repeated dose study of sucralose tolerance in human
    subjects. Food Chemical Toxicology. 38. Supplement 2.

S123-S129. 2000.

18. Goldsmith LA. Acute and subchronic toxicity of sucralose. Food Chemical Toxicology, 38. Supplement 2. S53-S69. 2000.

19. Mann S. W., Yuschak, M. M., Amyes, S. J. G., Aughton, P., & Finn, J. P. (2000a). A carcinogenicity study of sucralose in the CD-1 mouse. *Food Chemical Toxicology, 38* (Supplement 2), S99-S106.

20. Mann S. W., Yuschak, M. M., Amyes, S. J. G., Aughton, P. & Finn, J. P. (2000b). A combined chronic toxicity / carcinogenicity study of sucralose in Sprague-Dawley rats. *Food Chemical Toxicology, 38* (Supplement 2), S71-S89.

21. Baird IM, Shephard NW, Merritt RJ, Hildick-Smith G. Repeated dose study of sucralose tolerance in human subjects. *Food Chemical Toxicology. 38.* Supplement 2. S123-S129. 2000.

22. Kille J. W., Tesh, J. M., McAnulty, P. A., Ross, F. W., Willoughby, C. R., Bailey, G. P., Wilby, O. K. & Tesh, S. A. (2000). Sucralose: assessment of teratogenic potential in the rat and rabbit. *Food Chemical Toxicology, 38* (Supplement 2), S42-S52.

23. McNeil Speciality. (1998). Splenda (promotional information from McNeil Specialty Products Company).

24. Wood S. G., John B. A., & Hawkins, D. R. (2000). The pharmacokinetics and metabolism of sucralose in the dog. *Food Chemical Toxicology, 38* (Supplement 2), S99-S106.

25. John B. A., Wood S. G., & Hawkins, D. R. (2000a). The pharmacokinetics and metabolism of sucralose in the

mouse. *Food Chemical Toxicology, 38* (Supplement 2), S107-S110.

26. Roberts A., Renwick, A. G., Sims, J., & Snodin, D. J. (2000). Sucralose metabolism and pharmacokinetics in man. *Food Chemical Toxicology, 38* (Supplement 2), S31-S41.

27. John B. A., Wood, S. G., & Hawkins, D. R. (2000b). The pharmacokinetics and metabolism of sucralose in the rabbit. *Food Chemical Toxicology, 38* (Supplement 2), S111-S113.

28. Mezitis N. H. E., Maggio, C. A., Kock, P., Quddoos, A., Allison, D. B., & Pi-Sunyer, X. F. (1996). Glycemic effect of a single high oral dose of the novel sweetener sucralose in patients with diabetes. *Diabetes Care, 19,* 1004-1005.

29. Article Food and Chemical Toxicology. Volume 38. Supplement 2. Pages 123-129. Baird McLean, Shephard NW, Merrittc R., Hildick-Smith G. Medical Science Research: a Pine Court. Fairbourne, Cobham, Surrey KT11 2BT, UK. b Brambles. Granborough, Bucks, MK18 3NT, UK. c McNeil Specialty Products Company. 501 George St, New Brunswick, NJ 08903, USA. d Johnson & Johnson. World Tower. One Plaza, New Brunswick, NJ 08903. USA. Available online July 6, 2000. http://www.ncbi.nlm.nih.gov/entrez/query.fcgi?cmd=Retrieve&db=pubmed&dopt=Abstract&list_uids=10882825

30. The American Chemical Society. CAS division. Chlorinated sucrose sweeteners. International patent classification A23L001-236.

31. NIOSH. The National Institute for Occupational Safety and Health NIOSH is part of the Centers for Disease

References

Control and Prevention (CDC) in the Department of Health and Human Services.

32. Mann S. W., Yuschak, M. M., Amyes, S. J. G., Aughton, P. & Finn, J. P. (2000b). A combined chronic toxicity / carcinogenicity study of sucralose in Sprague-Dawley rats. *Food Chemical Toxicology, 38* (Supplement 2), S71-S89.

33. Grant D.L. Toxicological Evaluation Division Health and Welfare Canada. (Condensed. For the entire research report, visit the following link: http://europa.eu.int/comm/food/fs/sc/scf/out68_en.pdf

Sources Of Additional Information:

http://www.ncbi.nlm.nih.gov/entrez/query.fcgi for additional government studies

Barndt R. L., & Jackson, G. (1990). Stability of sucralose in baked goods. *Food Technology, 44,* 62-66.

Finn J P and Lord G H. Neurotoxicity studies on sucralose and its hydrolysis products with special reference to histopathologic and ultrastructural changes. Food Chemical Toxicology. 38 (Supplement 2), S7-S17. 2000.

Holder M. D., & Yirmiya, R. (1989). Behavioral assessment of the toxicity of aspartame. *Pharmacology Biochemistry Behavior, 32,* 17-26.

Lichtenthaler F. W., & Immel, S. (1999). Sucrose, sucralose, fructose, and some non-carbohydrate high-potency sweeteners: correlations between hydrophobicity patterns and AH-B-X assignments. *Sweet Taste Chemoreception, 21-53.*

Nabors L. O., & Gelardi, R. C. (1991). *Alternative Sweeteners,* Second edition. New York: Marcel Dekker, Inc., p. 194.

Quinlan M., Mialon, V., & Everitt, M. (1999). Effect of storage on the flavours of cola drinks sweetened with different sweetener systems. *World Rev. Nutrition Diet, 85,* 58-63.

Schiffman S. S., Sattely-Miller, E. A., Grahm, B. G., Bennett, J. L., Booth, B. J., Desai, N., & Bishay, I. (2000). Effect of temperature, pH, and ions on sweet taste. *Psychology & Behavior, 68,* 469-481.

Sims J., Roberts, A., Daniel, J. W. & Renwick, A. G. (2000). The metabolic fate of sucralose in rats. *Food Chemical Toxicology, 38* (Supplement 2), S115-S121.

Walters D. E. Sucralose. http://www.finchcms.edu/biochem/walters/sweet/sucralose.html. Viewed 10 April, 2001.

Wiet S. G., & Miller, G. A. (1997). Does chemical modification of tastants merely enhance their intrinsic taste qualitites? *Food Chemistry, 58*(4), 305-311.

Wood S. G., John, B. A., & Hawkins, D. R. (2000). The pharmacokinetics and metabolism of sucralose in the dog. *Food Chemical Toxicology, 38* (Supplement 2), S99-S106.

Yost D. A. (1989). Clinical safety of aspartame. *AFP, 39,* 201-205 (REVIEW).

http://www.ncbi.nlm.nih.gov/entrez/query.fcgi?CMD=Search&DB=pubmed:Flamm WG, Blackburn GL, Comer CP, Mayhew DA, Stargel WW. Long-term food consumption and body weight changes in neotame safety studies are consistent with the allometric relationship observed for other sweeteners and during dietary restrictions. Regul Toxicol Pharmacol. 2003

References

Oct;38(2):144-56. PMID: 14550756

Farhadi A, Keshavarzian A, Holmes EW, Fields J, Zhang L, Banan A. Gas chromatographic method for detection of urinary sucralose: application to the assessment of intestinal permeability. J Chromatogr B Analyt Technol Biomed Life Sci. 2003 Jan 25;784(1):145-54. PMID: 12504193

Mandel ID, Grotz VL.Dental considerations in sucralose use. J Clin Dent. 2002;13(3):116-8. PMID: 11887514

Bachmanov AA, Tordoff MG, Beauchamp GK. Sweetener preference of C57BL/6ByJ and 129P3/J mice. Chem Senses. 2001 Sep;26(7):905-13. PMID: 11555485

Nikolelis DP, Pantoulias S. A minisensor for the rapid screening of sucralose based on surface-stabilized bilayer lipid membranes. Biosens Bioelectron. 2000;15(9-10):439-44. PMID: 11419638 [PubMed - indexed for MEDLINE]

Baird IM, Shephard NW, Merritt RJ, Hildick-Smith G. Repeated dose study of sucralose tolerance in human subjects. Food Chem Toxicol. 2000;38 Suppl 2:S123-9. PMID: 10882825

Mann SW, Yuschak MM, Amyes SJ, Aughton P, Finn JP. A combined chronic toxicity/carcinogenicity study of sucralose in Sprague-Dawley rats. Food Chem Toxicol. 2000;38 Suppl 2: S71-89. PMID: 10882819

Goldsmith LA. Acute and subchronic toxicity of sucralose. Food Chem Toxicol. 2000;38 Suppl 2:S53-69. PMID: 10882818

Kille JW, Tesh JM, McAnulty PA, Ross FW, Willoughby CR, Bailey GP, Wilby OK, Tesh SA. Sucralose: assessment of teratogenic potential in the rat and the rabbit. Food Chem

Toxicol. 2000;38 Suppl 2:S43-52. PMID: 10882817

Kille JW, Ford WC, McAnulty P, Tesh JM, Ross FW, Willoughby CR. Sucralose: lack of effects on sperm glycolysis and reproduction in the rat. Food Chem Toxicol. 2000;38 Suppl 2:S19-29. PMID: 10882815

Finn JP, Lord GH. Neurotoxicity studies on sucralose and its hydrolysis products with special reference to histopathologic and ultrastructural changes. Food Chem Toxicol. 2000;38 Suppl 2:S7-17. PMID: 10882814

Mezitis NH, Maggio CA, Koch P, Quddoos A, Allison DB, Pi-Sunyer FX. Glycemic effect of a single high oral dose of the novel sweetener sucralose in patients with diabetes. Diabetes Care. 1996 Sep;19(9):1004-5. PMID: 8875098

Lord GH, Newberne PM. Renal mineralization--a ubiquitous lesion in chronic rat studies. Food Chem Toxicol. 1990 Jun;28(6):449-55. Review. PMID: 2210518

Edgar WM, Dodds MW. The effect of sweeteners on acid production in plaque. Int Dent J. 1985 Mar;35(1):18-22. PMID: 3858227

Department of Health & Human Services
http://www.ncbi.nlm.nih.gov/entrez/query.fcgi?CMD=Search&DB=pubmed

Hill AM, Belsito DV. Systemic contact dermatitis of the eyelids caused by formaldehyde derived from aspartame? Contact Dermatitis. 2003 Nov;49(5):258-9. No abstract available. PMID: 14996049

Van Wymelbeke V, Beridot-Therond ME, de La Gueronniere V, Fantino M. Influence of repeated consumption of beverages containing sucrose or intense sweeteners on food intake. Eur J Clin Nutr. 2004 Jan;58(1):154-61. PMID: 14679381

Hall WL, Millward DJ, Rogers PJ, Morgan LM. Physiological mechanisms mediating aspartame-induced satiety. Physiol Behav. 2003 Apr;78(4-5):557-62. PMID: 12782208

Vermunt SH, Pasman WJ, Schaafsma G, Kardinaal AF. Effects of sugar intake on body weight: a review. Obes Rev. 2003 May;4(2):91-9. Review. PMID: 12760444

Ilback NG, Alzin M, Jahrl S, Enghardt-Barbieri H, Busk L. Estimated intake of the artificial sweeteners acesulfame-K, aspartame, cyclamate and saccharin in a group of Swedish diabetics. Food Addit Contam. 2003 Feb;20(2):99-114. PMID: 12623659

Ottinger H, Soldo T, Hofmann T. Discovery and structure determination of a novel Maillard-derived sweetness enhancer by application of the comparative taste dilution analysis (cTDA). J Agric Food Chem. 2003 Feb 12;51(4):1035-41. PMID: 12568569

Nakamura T, Tanigake A, Miyanaga Y, Ogawa T, Akiyoshi T, Matsuyama K, Uchida T. The effect of various substances on the suppression of the bitterness of quinine-human gustatory sensation, binding, and taste sensor studies. Chem Pharm Bull (Tokyo). 2002 Dec;50(12):1589-93. PMID: 12499596

Shannon M. An empathetic look at overweight. CCL Family Found. 1993 Nov-Dec;20(3):3, 5. PMID: 12318598

Butchko HH, Stargel WW, Comer CP, Mayhew DA, Benninger C, Blackburn GL, de Sonneville LM, Geha RS, Hertelendy Z, Koestner A, Leon AS, Liepa GU, McMartin KE, Mendenhall CL, Munro IC, Novotny EJ, Renwick AG, Schiffman SS,

Schomer DL, Shaywitz BA, Spiers PA, Tephly TR, Thomas JA, Trefz FK. Aspartame: review of safety. Regul Toxicol Pharmacol. 2002 Apr;35(2 Pt 2):S1-93. Review. PMID: 12180494

Laffort P, Walsh RM, Spillane WJ. Application of the U and gamma' models in binary sweet taste mixtures. Chem Senses. 2002 Jul;27(6):511-20. PMID: 12142327

Aires CP, Tabchoury CP, Del Bel Cury AA, Cury JA. Effect of a lactose-containing sweetener on root dentine demineralization in situ. Caries Res. 2002 May-Jun;36(3):167-9. PMID: 12065968

Sunram-Lea SI, Foster JK, Durlach P, Perez C. Investigation into the significance of task difficulty and divided allocation of resources on the glucose memory facilitation effect. Psychopharmacology (Berl). 2002 Apr;160(4):387-97. Epub 2002 Feb 08. PMID: 11919666

Schulz KF, Grimes DA. Sample size slippages in randomised trials: exclusions and the lost and wayward. Lancet. 2002 Mar 2;359(9308):781-5. PMID: 11888606

Zheng JY, Fulu MY, Lee DY, Barber TE, Adjei AL. Pulmonary peptide delivery: effect of taste-masking excipients on leuprolide suspension metered-dose inhalers. Pharm Dev Technol. 2001 Nov;6(4):521-30. PMID: 11775953

Ouwens MJ, Tan FE, Berger MP. Local influence to detect influential data structures for generalized linear mixed models. Biometrics. 2001 Dec;57(4):1166-72. PMID: 11764257

Weihrauch MR, Diehl V, Bohlen H. [Artificial sweeteners--are they potentially carcinogenic?] Med Klin (Munich). 2001 Nov 15;96(11):670-5. Review. German. Erratum in: Med Klin 2002

Mar 15;97(3):173. PMID: 11760654

Butchko HH, Stargel WW. Aspartame: scientific evaluation
in the postmarketing period. Regul Toxicol Pharmacol. 2001
Dec;34(3):221-33. PMID: 11754527

Sakai N, Kobayakawa T, Gotow N, Saito S, Imada S.
Enhancement of sweetness ratings of aspartame by a vanilla
odor presented either by orthonasal or retronasal routes.
Percept Mot Skills. 2001 Jun;92(3 Pt 2):1002-8. PMID:
11565908

Bachmanov AA, Tordoff MG, Beauchamp GK. Sweetener
preference of C57BL/6ByJ and 129P3/J mice. Chem Senses.
2001 Sep;26 (7):905-13. PMID: 11555485

Sunram-Lea SI, Foster JK, Durlach P, Perez C. Glucose
facilitation of cognitive performance in healthy young adults:
examination of the influence of fast-duration, time of day and
pre-consumption plasma glucose levels. Psychopharmacology
(Berl). 2001 Aug;157(1):46-54. PMID: 11512042

Chapter 9
Sneak Peeks Into Little-Known Sweetener Facts

http://www.financialexpress-bd.com/index3.asp?cnd=5/27/
2004&section_id=6&newsid=10861&spcl=no

http://www.cspinet.org/sodapop/liquid_candy.htm

http://www.nsda.org/SoftDrinks/

http://www.pregnancy.org/article.php?sid=890

http://www.blacktable.com/gillin040317.htm

http://www.ourstolenfuture.org/NewScience/reproduction/TDS/2001skakkebaeketal.htm

FDA Rules and Regulations **Federal Register** Report Vol. 63, No. 64

For more information on Did You Know Topics, visit the following links and reference sources:

http://www.financialexpress-bd.com/index3.asp?cnd=5/27/2004&section_id=6&newsid=10861&spcl=no

http://www.cspinet.org/sodapop/liquid_candy.htm

http://www.nsda.org/SoftDrinks/

http://www.pregnancy.org/article.php?sid=890

http://www.blacktable.com/gillin040317.htm

http://www.ourstolenfuture.org/NewScience/reproduction/TDS/2001skakkebaeketal.htm

Chapter 10
The Sweetener Wars

Hirsch JM. Should be, Diers may face Shortage: dieters may face Splenda shortage. Associated Press. December 2004.

Caruso DB. Maker of Equal Sues Marketer of Splenda. Associated Press. Philadelphia. Dec 1, 2004.

Hull JS. Sweet Poison: How The World's Most Popular Artificial Sweetener Is Killing Us-My Story. New Horizon Press, 1997.

References

Sources Of Additional Information:

Knight I. (1993). The development and applications of sucralose, a new high-intensity sweetener. *Canadian Journal of Physiology and Pharmacology, 72,* 435-439 (REVIEW).

McNeil Speciality. (1998). Splenda (promotional information from McNeil Specialty Products Company).

http://www.ajinomoto.ch Ajinomoto Switzerland AG

"Business Weekly", May 5, 2004.

"Coca-Cola's Low-Carb Soda Loses Its Fizz", Chad Terhune, *The Wall Street Journal*, Wednesday, October 20, 2004.

Mohl B. Boston Globe. February 22, 2005 http://www.sfgate.com/cgi-bin/article.cgi?file=/chronicle/archive/2005/02/22//chronicle/info/copyright/ ©2005 San Francisco Chronicle

http://www.aspartame.info/index.html

http://www.aspartame.info/aspartame/aspartame%20contact.asp
(http://www.brandchannel.com/features_effect.asp?id=155)

http://www.holisticmed.com/splenda/

http://www.monsanto.com/monsanto/layout/about_us/ataglance.asp

http://www.jnj.com/innovations/new_features/splenda.htm

http://www.chemindustry.com/chem2ask.asp?cmd=search